Appreciative Healthcare Practice

Full the full range of M&K Publishing books please visit our website:

www.mkupdate.co.uk

Appreciative Healthcare Practice

A guide to compassionate person-centred care

Gwilym Wyn Roberts and Andrew Machon

Appreciative Healthcare Practice: A guide to compassionate person-centres care

Gwilym Wyn Roberts and Andrew Machon

ISBN: 9781905539-93-2

First published 2015

All rights reserved. No part of this publication may be reproduced, stored in a retrieval system, or transmitted in any form or by any means, electronic, mechanical, photocopying, recording or otherwise, without either the prior permission of the publishers or a licence permitting restricted copying in the United Kingdom issued by the Copyright Licensing Agency, 90 Tottenham Court Road, London, WIT 4LP. Permissions may be sought directly from M&K Publishing, phone: 01768 773030, fax: 01768 781099 or email: publishing@mkupdate.co.uk

Any person who does any unauthorised act in relation to this publication may be liable to criminal prosecution and civil claims for damages.

British Library Cataloguing in Publication Data

A catalogue record for this book is available from the British Library

Notice

Clinical practice and medical knowledge constantly evolve. Standard safety precautions must be followed, but, as knowledge is broadened by research, changes in practice, treatment and drug therapy may become necessary or appropriate. Readers must check the most current product information provided by the manufacturer of each drug to be administered and verify the dosages and correct administration, as well as contraindications. It is the responsibility of the practitioner, utilising the experience and knowledge of the patient, to determine dosages and the best treatment for each individual patient. Any brands mentioned in this book are as examples only and are not endorsed by the publisher. Neither the publisher nor the authors assume any liability for any injury and/or damage to persons or property arising from this publication.

Disclaimer

M&K Publishing cannot accept responsibility for the contents of any linked website or online resource. The existence of a link does not imply any endorsement or recommendation of the organisation or the information or views which may be expressed in any linked website or online resource. We cannot guarantee that these links will operate consistently and we have no control over the availability of linked pages.

To contact M&K Publishing write to:
M&K Update Ltd · The Old Bakery · St. John's Street
Keswick · Cumbria CA12 5AS
Tel: 01768 773030 · Fax: 01768 781099
publishing@mkupdate.co.uk
www.mkupdate.co.uk

Designed and typeset by Mary Blood

Printed in Scotland by Bell & Bain Ltd.

Contents

Foreword *vii*
About the authors *viii*
Introduction *ix*
Personal stories *xiii*
    From daughter to carer *xiii*
    Being cared for after trauma *xiv*
    From carer to protector *xvi*
    Protector and advocate *xvii*

Chapter 1
Compassionate and dignified care *1*

Chapter 2
Professionalism – on becoming a professional *11*

Chapter 3
Problem-solving in healthcare *21*

Chapter 4
Applying appreciative inquiry in practice and education *31*

Chapter 5
Creativity and care *41*

Chapter 6
Applying the three-eye model to healthcare *53*

Chapter 7
Mindful healthcare practice *71*

Chapter 8
The appreciative care worker and coach *89*

Chapter 9
Conclusion *109*

References *115*
Bibliography *123*

Foreword

I believe this book may become one of the most important of our time for those of us in work that involves the care of others. The volume and type of demands and changes we face in caring work means we may lose our capacity to 'be' and care in the pressure to 'do', work and deliver. Open-hearted individuals wishing to care may face stress and an experience of burnout in the face of these demands. This book has a special gift in dealing with a complex subject that is hard to express in a way that is accessible to those that need to understand more fully. The book gives us the language and perspective that makes this subject communicable and one that can be taught, explored and learnt. The book also shows us a paradox: in care, appreciation and creativity we can find the best in us, give the best in us, care while delivering tasks that are asked of us, and at the same time care for ourselves. This book will help us find more of our own humanity as well as caring via that humanity.

Piers Worth PhD
Chartered Psychologist. Accredited Psychotherapist.
Reader in Psychology – Bucks New University

About the authors

Dr Gwilym Wyn Roberts

Senior Lecturer, Cardiff University EdD, MA, Diploma in Applied Psychosynthesis, Dip (COT)

Gwilym has worked at Cardiff University as Director of Occupational Therapy and Senior Lecturer since 2002. He is a registered Occupational Therapist and a qualified Applied Psychosynthesis Psychotherapist. He has a Master's degree in Further and Higher Education from the Institute of Education in London and a Professional Doctorate from the School of Social Sciences at Cardiff University. His main research interests are the enhancement of problem-based learning and the application of appreciative inquiry in practice and education. He is particularly interested in the patient's experience relating to compassion and dignity, and he sits on the Wales Crown Prosecution Hate Crime, Modern Slavery and Human Trafficking Panel. He has recently extended his research interests into the areas of elder abuse, mental health and palliative and end of life care.

Dr Andrew Machon

PhD, MA, BSc (Hons) Biochemistry

Andrew has a PhD in Biochemistry and has become a leading accredited executive business coach. He is a rare blend of scientist, artist, psychotherapist, teacher and author. Andrew has worked across the globe as an executive business coach and change specialist, consulting with major multinational organisations. Although he is a qualified psychosynthesis psychotherapist, his current practice is mainly focused on his work as a coach and coach supervisor. As an experienced coaching supervisor, he specialises in the professional and personal development of fellow coaches. Andrew also lectures on several subjects, including positive psychology and compassionate care, at both undergraduate and postgraduate levels in UK universities.

Introduction

'Caring is a sustained emotional investment in an individual's well-being characterised by a desire to take actions that will benefit that person.'
(Weiner & Auster 2007)

Why is this book needed?

Being a healthcare professional presupposes that we care. Yet there is plentiful evidence, most notably the Francis Report (2013), showing that carers can at times become uncaring, and professionals can become unprofessional and even be abusive to their clients. How can this happen? This is the vital question that has prompted us to write this book.

The reaction to such evidence of 'mis-care' is often to name and blame the isolated few. However, we propose that every health- and social care professional and support worker is capable of a spectrum of care, from total lack of care through to compassionate care. Placing blame outside ourselves removes our awareness of our own limitations and strengths as practitioners. It is human nature to be blind to our own blindness. Yet our ability to care for others largely depends on our ability to be self-aware, to self-manage and to self-care.

What are our aims?

In this book, we offer a model that enables healthcare workers to see the full scope of their potential practice. The 'three eyes' approach invites practitioners to look at their caring practice from three different perspectives: the analytical, the appreciative and the creative. Each of these 'eyes' provides a particular view of caring and offers the practitioner specific skills and qualities to bring to their practice.

This book invites us all to work more consciously, to continually expand our awareness and vision in order to appreciate fully what it means to be a carer. In exploring the analytical eye, we gain insight into what it may mean to mis-care for our clients. In learning how to open an appreciative eye, we examine the importance of mindfulness in healthcare practice. And as we continue to develop and grow as reflective practitioners, we automatically become better at including and engaging our clients. By opening the creative eye, we can examine what it means to be a truly conscious, person-centred and responsive carer and learn how to show compassion and dignity through our practice.

A central principle we examine is that our 'lock' is also our 'key'. In other words, we have to develop our insight in order to see how we may reactively (and often quite unconsciously) mis-care. Becoming aware of how we can sometimes limit and lock away our potential as carers is key to developing best practice. Essentially, becoming a compassionate and dignified practitioner means learning how to open new eyes on the way we care.

As we learn how to access these three eyes, we gain particular skills and qualities that enable us to become healthcare coaches as well as practitioners. Through coaching conversations in our everyday work, we can see the client beyond their diagnosis and enable them to become more actively involved in their own care. Despite the challenge of illness and adversity, the opportunity is there for any healthcare practitioner to draw out what the client needs and desires, in line with the client's own values, purposes and beliefs. This approach seeks to alleviate suffering and allows the client to be more empowered and motivated to change, discovering choice and possibility in times of potential adversity. The practitioner therefore not only enables the client to self-manage and self-care but also helps them to increase their own resilience and resourcefulness.

Another central theme of this book is that, to care for another, we first have to learn how to care for ourselves. How we develop self-care is a vital consideration for the healthcare practitioner who intends to sustain best practice. We sincerely hope that readers of this book (whether they are healthcare workers, healthcare students, support workers, carers or clients or anyone with an interest in dignified and compassionate care) will find it useful and informative. We also hope that it will encourage readers to make a lifelong commitment to skill development and reflection in order to achieve an exemplary level of care for themselves and naturally therefore for others.

Our intention is that every reader will gain insight and deepen their awareness of what it means to be a person-centred and responsive carer, to experience what it means to bring 'your best self' to your work and daily caring practice. Thus, for example, 'the hip in the corner' or 'bed 7 needs a commode' will become 'Catherine who has had a hip replacement' or 'Mr Patel needs a commode'. By caring for people as individual human beings we learn to respect each other's originality and value and offer dignified, respectful practice.

Illness often leaves people feeling vulnerable, disempowered, confused and dependent on the expertise of others. What greater act of service is there than to help a client re-find their own compass and sense of direction? It is vital for anyone in this situation to realise that they can discover opportunity in adversity, find meaning in their lives, be resourceful and continue to grow and develop, despite the challenges of illness. Indeed, this realisation may be key to health, well-being and healing.

Introduction

How is the book structured?

We begin with a selection of personal stories, which motivated us to write this book and provide some real-life context. After this, the book is divided into two halves. In Chapters 1–5, we discuss in detail the current challenges and emerging opportunities for carers. In Chapters 6–8, we look at the development and application of the skills and qualities of the healthcare worker, and how responsive person-centred practice can be realised and sustained.

Chapter 1 explores existing evidence of uncaring practice, and highlights the aspirations of healthcare practitioners and what it means to work with compassion and dignity.

Chapter 2 looks at the complex requirements of working as a healthcare professional and, in contrast, the characteristics of unprofessional practice.

Chapter 3 examines the usual approach to problem-solving in healthcare practice and introduces the first part of our three-eye model – the analytical eye. We illustrate how the problem-solving impulse can sometimes limit the vision of the student and practitioner.

Chapter 4 introduces the second eye of our model – the appreciative eye – along with an appreciation of what it means to be a more reflective, empathic practitioner

Chapter 5 explores the nature of creativity in education and practice and illustrates how opening the third eye of our model – the creative eye – can lead to a more person-centred practice that releases the client's true potential.

Chapter 6 explains the three-eye model in more detail and looks at the relationship between the analytical, appreciative and creative eyes, and how each offers a characteristic vision and approach to caring.

Chapter 7 examines the importance of developing a more mindful practice and how this can inform more responsive, person-centred care.

Chapter 8 develops the concept of the appreciative healthcare worker as a coach. We show how the coaching approach can help the client foster their own well-being and feel motivated to self-manage and self-care, despite the challenges of ill health.

Who is this book for?

Throughout the book, we consider both the student–tutor relationship and the practitioner–client relationship, and focus on both healthcare education and healthcare practice. The book should therefore provide a valuable learning resource for a wide range of individuals involved in caring practices. Whatever your particular role or situation, we hope it will offer you insight, support and guidance in becoming a more compassionate carer.

A note on terminology

For the sake of consistency, we have used the term 'client' to refer to patients, service users and all individuals who find themselves in the position of being cared for. We have used the term 'healthcare' to mean all settings and organisations with responsibility for providing such care. These organisations include the statutory services provided by the National Health Service and local authority/social services as well as those run by the private and/or the voluntary sector. Finally, we have used the term 'care worker' to represent a broad cross-section of individuals who work in health- and social care. These may include highly qualified and regulated professional practitioners, healthcare and medical students, support staff and any individuals who find themselves on the front line of caring for sick and vulnerable people.

Personal stories

The following real-life stories have been shared by individuals who have experienced different levels of care (either personally or affecting a vulnerable family member), ranging from kind and compassionate to uncompassionate, undignified and at times abusive. In addition to reports identifying uncaring and often abusive practice that we reference throughout, including the Francis Report (2013) and the Baker Report (2011), we wanted to include some personal stories that came to our attention whilst writing this book.

These personal experiences bring home the scale of the challenge for the reader. They set the context for the book and they have motivated us to develop a model that shows: firstly how the practice of any care worker can become uncaring and times abusive; and secondly how, based on this insight, we can learn to foster compassionate, person-centred care.

Some professionals may question the content of some of these stories but they are described by the individual contributors as they experienced them in real life. These and other personal accounts motivated the writing of this book.

From daughter to carer

From a very early age until the day I left home, I remember my clothes moving from the floor in my bedroom to being washed, ironed and back in the wardrobe. It was a miracle – it was my mum.

On 27 February 2013 my world and my relationship with mum was to change forever. It was the day she was diagnosed with acute myeloid leukemia (AML). Mum had been tired and had poor blood results for some time until a consultant she was referred to asked for a bone marrow check to determine exactly what was wrong. This consultant was very assertive, yet kind, gave time and showed compassion to my mum in her distress. He became the man who would hold the key to my mum's destiny. From that day onwards, our diary was no longer social trips and late night shopping but full of medical appointments and stays in hospital for chemotherapy and the day unit for blood and platelet transfusions.

I never thought that the concept of the 'parent–child' approach would be used by me and Mum once she was diagnosed with cancer. I have become the parent and Mum has become the child… In Macmillan terms, I am now classed as 'a carer'. As a carer, but more importantly as a daughter, I have had to watch my mum being transformed from a strong, proud and lively woman to a lady who is grateful for every moment of care and compassion that she receives. My mum is very proud and has a lot of dignity.

Healthcare must be a difficult world to be in. I have seen excellent and caring doctors, nurses and therapists and sadly I have also witnessed those who are not. To some professionals, my mum was just a number above a bed, on a board or on a chart. We have had a situation where one nurse referred to a patient as 'bed 6 needs her catheter changed'. There are times I have wanted to shout, 'That's my mum you're sticking needles into, talking about her as if she is deaf, leaving her in bed with just a tad of dignity. If it was your mum, would you treat her like you treat mine?'

As Mum accepts that she needs her treatment to try to keep her alive, she also acknowledges the fine care she is given and sees the anguish of others in a similar position to her. Unfortunately not everyone is the same. One evening Mum was unwell after going to the day centre. She had a blood transfusion, following which she was discharged at 9pm. Mum got to the entrance of the hospital and felt unwell. I decided to return her to the ward, as I was fearful that her temperature was so high and there would be a risk of infection. We were met by a junior doctor. He took our details and Mum's temperature and said it wasn't high enough to admit her. I experienced him as rude and dismissive, showing no compassion or dignity to myself or Mum. I took Mum home that night, only to return two hours later, when Mum was admitted with a severe infection.

On reflection, I believe that illness and heartache go hand in hand. But it makes life more bearable when you are helped by doctors, therapists and nurses who really care, who show compassion, treat you with dignity, and see you as a person and not as a statistic. Those professionals are out there. My mum's consultant, for example, is authoritative but kind and takes time to see his patients, regardless of a heavy list. He has always made Mum feel as if she is his most important patient.

All we want is a caring professional who is willing to listen and show compassion and treat us with dignity. I need someone I can trust when I have to leave Mum on the ward or unit. It costs nothing to be kind, to hold a hand and offer reassurance. It does make a big difference to patients and loved ones when they are at their most vulnerable! It's not our choice to be in the hospital or day unit, but it is a choice for professional staff to work there!

KAW, Cardiff

Being cared for after trauma

I was an apparently healthy, professional man who exercised regularly. I used to run half-marathon races and I did this partly for fun and partly to raise money for charities. In November 2014, I went for a 12km run before making breakfast on a Sunday morning. About halfway round, I realised that I was having a stroke. I had lost all the function on the left-hand side of my body. I tried to stand up but kept falling into the brambles and nettles beside the road. After a lot of struggling, I managed to get myself to a nearby house. There was no one in so I tried to get to the next house, and then had a second stroke that filled my head with blood and stopped me completely.

I had only a quarter vision left in my right eye, and it was like looking down a tunnel. I lay by the road in the brambles and nettles. Fortunately a man and then a couple came along and found me. They called for an ambulance, which took me to hospital. At that point I passed out. When I came to, after several hours, I could hear (but not see) my wife. I realised I had lost all movement on the left-hand side of my body and had very limited vision.

My consciousness of caring started in the hospital. I was in the highly critical ward and the staff were very concerned. They tried to communicate with me, and I with them, but it was impossible to have a meaningful conversation. I was in fact very frightened and for the first five days I didn't go to sleep because I was scared that I would not wake up again.

After a while, the carers gave me confidence that I could trust in them and that I could have a proper rest, but it was very traumatic. I woke up early one morning, covered in blood, and I had pulled some of the tubes out of my arm. Two young nurses came and very tenderly bathed me and removed the blood and dressed me again and rolled me back into the bed. I was amazed by the tender, kind way they treated me when I was in such a horrible mess.

My memories of kindness range from people bringing me a drink to one of the therapists coming to massage my body to get some feeling back in my arms and my legs. One memory that stands out very strongly was the time when three therapists took on the task of trying to get my legs moving again. It actually took three of them to lift me up and make me take eight steps across the ward. At the end of those eight steps we were all utterly shattered. It was mostly them making my legs move but what a tremendous sense they gave me of real progress, achievement and success.

All the levels I went through, from the very extreme care to the point where they signed me off to a different hospital and rehabilitation, to support to be at home, I felt the carers did more than they were paid to do. At first, I could only move with a frame with four wheels on but they had a plan to get me home and to be able to do all that I would need to do. Could I make toast and make a cup of coffee? Could I learn words? One of them would take me to the exercise area; another one would check if I had practised my words and would stay and help.

Everyone to me seemed to have their own particular kindness and gentleness and I was touched by that. For instance, one nurse heard me say that I hated the hospital coffee and she used to prepare me a hot chocolate at bedtime. Another nurse, who seemed severe, was always stretching and pushing me. For example, it was she who got me to be able to shower on my own. This was very affirming and made me feel more self-sufficient. Each carer, in their way, was very faithful in caring for me – was dedicated to me. I feel they saw me as a person beyond my condition. I think they were responding to me and what I needed. I did notice there was a divide in the rehabilitation group. Some patients had given up hope and I imagine it must be more difficult to do something positive to help someone in that frame of mind. From the start, I was determined that I was going to do something to improve my situation. I am guessing that it's easier to care for someone who is responding positively.

My care continued into my home, where I set up on the ground floor. A combination of nurses and therapists worked with me, getting me upstairs to have a shower and helping me get back into normal family life. I had six weeks of this intensive help, which I valued enormously.

Finally, let me say something about the hospital. It was apparently failing but it has had more attention over the last few years. It now has better staffing levels and appears to be beating local targets, from what I understand. There seems to be a common philosophy amongst all the staff, whether in intensive care or rehabilitation or home support. They all work as one team.

FC, Worcester

From carer to protector

My mother was diagnosed with Alzheimer's in 2008. She was sectioned under the Mental Health Act and we were not given any information about her condition or the process or the contacts. I was advised by mobile telephone by the psychiatrist that my mother had Alzheimer's. After four weeks of visiting the hospital, she found the environment very frightening and intimidating. Not once did anyone update my brother or myself and therefore we requested a meeting with the Healthcare Authority to express some of our concerns.

In the end we duly found a care home, and my mother was there for about two years. We visited regularly but one day we arrived unannounced, only to find her in her room in soiled clothing and bedding, dehydrated and distressed. The care home had also mislaid her teeth, glasses and personal clothing. We moved her to a new home, due to the neglect that she received in the first care home!

When she was hospitalised she was kept on a trolley for three days in A & E because they did not have a bed. She was admitted later on to another hospital, due to dehydration. On her return to the care home, I was advised that a DNR ('do not resuscitate') had been applied to my mother's care notes. At no point was this discussed with either my brother or myself.

We attended a case review at the care home to discuss nursing care support. The person assessing my mother's needs did not even go and look at my mother and ran through a checklist which I thought was clearly weighted to refuse support. My mother was 80 years old and unable to communicate, could not move, could not communicate her needs, was doubly incontinent, and had to be fed and constantly attended to. She weighed under 6 stone and yet did not qualify for CHC (continuing healthcare)!

Some professional staff showed no sign of empathy or sympathy towards my mother, brother or myself and decisions were taken without consultation or communication. My mother's life savings of £50,000 were spent on her care and we are now accruing a debt over her house to fund my mother's care… And the story goes on.

JP, Bedfordshire

Protector and advocate

Let me introduce my mum, Ingrid. She was intelligent, kind, feisty and a loyal friend. Not having enjoyed a stable childhood herself, when Ingrid became a mother at 35 years old, she and Ted (my dad) made a priority of providing a stable and loving home. Mum set herself the task of being the best mother she could be, and she worked selflessly to give us the best upbringing she could. Food was always freshly cooked, education was high on the agenda as she and my dad wanted opportunities for us they never had themselves, and she took a series of part-time jobs to fit in with school hours to provide many activities for us. Mum was a fierce supporter of her children in every way but we had a lot of fun and music often filled the house. Sadly she became very disabled at 55 years of age, due to severe rheumatoid arthritis. As a sufferer of the same disease myself, I now know first-hand why her doctors called her 'stoic'. Although her mobility was limited, she bore the stiffness, constant exhaustion and pain with little complaint.

Mum was diagnosed with Alzheimer's in 2007 when she came to live with us, following the death of my dad. It was clear by then that the disease had been advancing for some time and Dad had clearly made the decision to keep these worries to himself, a pact with Mum if you like. They had been together 57 years at this point, and inseparable, so that was not surprising.

We had the good fortune of having a supportive family who were brilliant about providing us with respite breaks, but caring for someone with this disease is a hard and upsetting rollercoaster for everyone. Many people think dementia is simply about becoming more forgetful. It is surely one of the cruellest afflictions, with sufferers losing first all the memories, both happy and sad, that provide the continuity and richness in all our lives, and then losing themselves. Fear and anger were regular visitors to Mum during this horrendous process. As a carer, grief and loss are constant, as the person you know and love gradually disappears but is still physically present, with ever-increasing needs to be met.

Most of the health professionals we encountered were sympathetic but totally unable to provide anything like acceptable services and support. I was very alone and felt that I had to find my own way through all of it. An Occupational Therapist visited our home to assess whether we qualified for any building work or equipment for Mum. She completed her assessment by saying 'I hope you know what you are letting yourself in for.' Very helpful.

The best help I received in the community was through the Alzheimer's Society, who put me in touch with Crossroads, who provided help for carers. They became my guardian angels over the next five years.

I would not have missed this precious time with my mum. I miss her still. People asked how I could keep going. I genuinely had no wish or desire to do otherwise. Then the second worst day of my life to date came when I realised that Mum's condition had deteriorated to an extent beyond my personal capability to go on caring for her, as she needed 24/7 nursing care. My husband was having to do more than was reasonable to help and I had my own health issues to deal with. I had to find a nursing home.

The search for a home good enough for my mum was soul-destroying. The Care Quality Commission's grading system was pitiful at that point. What they graded as 'satisfactory' or 'good' was so far from that in my eyes. Most places say they provide dementia care but they do not. This should not be allowed under the Trades Descriptions Act, as the majority mean they can only cope with those who have moderate dementia. I asked what would happen if my mum called out for attention at night (something which at that point happened regularly). One care home manager said that she might disturb other residents, another said she could press a button to call staff – Mum couldn't even answer a ringing phone at this point, let alone remember what a buzzer was for! The majority of care homes I visited were in a poor state of repair and the CQC seemed to have no power to press owners to bring them up to a good standard. They may have been clean but they were grim. Also, it soon became clear that if the dementia became more severe we would have to find another home.

Staff may be kind, but providing more than adequate care for someone with severe dementia takes so much more. I was clear that Mum needed to make this move only once. Anything else would not be in her best interest so my search continued for a home that provided both full nursing and dementia specialist care. Finally I found a newly completed dementia specialist home, which was 30 minutes from my home, and a manager who I felt I could work with. The home promised outings (unlike most places I visited) and nursing-led care, and the staff were well trained and – above all – person-centred care was high on the agenda. It was still the worst day of my life when I had to leave Mum there. The upheaval alone affected Mum for at least six to nine months. I felt nothing but guilt and sadness.

I have personal experience of dealing with the complex, highly individual needs of a severe dementia sufferer. It requires training, resourcefulness, limitless understanding and compassion in situations where the person to be cared for may be aggressive, annoying, highly repetitive in demands or actions, so scared they shout for help constantly or with little or no communication at all. How do you know the person is ill or in pain if they can't tell you? How can they be tempted to eat? What do you need to do to keep the person feeling safe, occupied, etc.? Has a person's behaviour changed? Does this mean they are unwell or just entering another phase of the dementia? And finally, of course, how do you deal with death in a dignified way?

In addition to all this, care home staff are often dealing with multiple other conditions that come with age. I found this a challenge myself, as a relatively well-educated, caring person.

So, what was the care home experience like? Initially the home had some management problems, which meant that promises of exceptional care were not delivered, but now things are much improved. Fundamentally, what is asked of staff here on a daily basis and what they are paid do not match up to the responsibility of providing dignified, compassionate person-centred care.

Consistency for me is at the heart of high-quality care. But the reality is that staff are often on 12-hour shifts, with minimum wage for carers and significant management responsibilities for the nurses. There is a constant battle to keep staff – a turnover of 30% per annum is seen as acceptable. So things just seem to settle down and then the best people often leave, followed by yet another round of mistakes and learning as new staff members get up to speed. With Alzheimer's, knowing the individual is central to care-giving, so staff turnover impacts negatively on all care home residents, who are some of the most vulnerable people in our society.

Training is given in Mum's care home, which is good, but the full effect is limited by constant staff changes. The people who care for Mum and the other residents look after them as well as they can and do want to do their best. I have not come across anyone who did not want to do their best, but sadly this doesn't mean that care is always good or acceptable. For me, this means constant vigilance and a struggle to ensure that Mum gets what she needs. It is exhausting.

We should ask a lot of people who work in care homes. Our elders deserve dignified, respectful care and compassion at all times, to their very last breath. Acceptable (not minimum) standards of training, pay and working hours should provide a framework in which care is delivered and local authorities should ensure the fees they pay allow these standards to be met – not set at a minimum level. Not just anyone can be a carer; it is a tiring, complex, difficult job, where death and dying are part of life on a daily basis. Why then in hourly pay terms is it equated with an unskilled production line task?

Mum is now increasingly frail, bedridden and cannot move. She cannot communicate her needs at all or speak, and is doubly incontinent. All feeding and drinking has to be managed for her, she has a purée diet and swallowing issues mean it can take over an hour to get minimal meals finished. She has to be washed and dressed. Her skin is so fragile – even leaving a creased bed sheet can cause an irritation, which could result in bed sores. She has advanced congestive heart failure and is prone to chest and urine infections that can become serious very quickly. Mum's remaining pleasures are having her hand held and listening to music. She is generally cared for well by people who, on the whole, despite their pay and conditions, are dedicated, caring and compassionate in what they do, but this takes a lot of continuous effort to achieve.

Finally we heard that Mum qualified for Continuing Healthcare, as she has been declared 'at end of life'. We appear to be lucky, as many don't get the award until after their relative dies.

Abraham Joshua Herschel said: 'A test of a people is how it behaves toward the old. It is easy to love children. Even tyrants and dictators make a point of being fond of children. But the affection and care for the old, the incurable, the helpless are the true gold mines of a culture.'

On this basis, our culture is in trouble and things need to change quickly to ensure that all the elderly and infirm receive the real compassion, dignity and standards of care they deserve, and caring becomes a profession that is revered and rewarded accordingly. Only then will relatives not have to fight a constant war against an unjust system.

JJ, London

Chapter 1

Compassionate and dignified care

Introduction

This chapter describes some of the policies and legislation that have focused on compassion and dignity in health- and social care. Recent policy documents and acts of parliament have tried to move away from the paternalistic model, in which practitioners 'do things to' people, in favour of a more proactive, interactive approach, in which clients play a bigger role in their own care. In this chapter we also discuss our understanding of what it means to be caring and to be cared for, the nature of the caring relationship and its effects, and the impact of situations when things go drastically wrong, and clients and colleagues are let down by a lack of basic standards and awareness. Engaging individuals in their own health and care is now recognised as a major component in developing a health service of the highest quality.

The delivery of effective, competent, safe client care has to be a priority for all healthcare organisations and governments (Kirwan *et al.* 2013, Najjar *et al.* 2013, Pinder *et al.* 2013, Dixon-Woods 2013). In the UK, there is no doubt that the vast majority of healthcare professionals and support workers (including those in the private and voluntary sectors) are dedicated to delivering excellent care services in a dignified and compassionate environment. Most aspire to meet each client's physical, mental, emotional and spiritual needs from a place of dedication and commitment. Upholding the core values of excellence, dignity, justice, collaboration and stewardship serves not just clients, but colleagues, organisations and society in general.

Nevertheless, despite a wide range of quality initiatives and a string of high-profile policies and targets focused specifically on delivering compassion and dignity in health and social care, there is substantial evidence that these aspects are still being compromised (Care Quality Commission 2011, Francis Report 2013, Andrews Report 2014). Notably,

The Operating Framework for the NHS in England 2012–13. (DH 2011) aimed to prioritise the care of vulnerable adults, and in particular older adults. This Framework stated clearly that parts of the NHS were failing to provide dignified and compassionate care or to offer acceptable standards in areas such as continence, nutrition and communication. In 2011, the Parliamentary and Health Service Ombudsman reported 10 cases of older adults who died unnecessarily after being admitted to NHS hospitals. Alarmingly, most did not receive what society would consider the most basic standards of care, such as easy access to drinking water. The publication of such reports and policies is crucial, as they provide the impetus to push for faster improvement in quality of care.

The Keogh (2013), Berwick (2013), Andrews (2014) and in particular the Francis (2013) reports have highlighted the key role that all professionals, support workers and indeed healthcare students have to play in delivering high-quality, compassionate and dignified person-centred care. We mention students here because the Francis Report's many recommendations included the proposal that undergraduate nursing programmes should give students practical experience in delivering competent, compassionate care (pp. 1539–40). The Nursing and Midwifery Council (NMC) responded that this recommendation would be met through revised education standards predating the inquiry. It remains to be seen if and how it will indeed be met.

The Francis Report, 2013

In evaluating current health and social care, the ability to understand and appraise any policy, procedure or legislation is vital, as it encourages evidence-based professional practice (Upton *et al.* 2014). In 2010, the then Secretary of State for Health, Andrew Lansley MP, announced a full public inquiry into the role of the commissioning, supervisory and regulatory bodies who monitored work within the Mid Staffordshire NHS Foundation Trust. The Francis Report, which emerged from this inquiry, has become one of the most significant and influential reports focusing on compassion and dignity.

According to the Francis Report, up to 1,200 people died unnecessarily in appalling circumstances in Mid Staffordshire NHS Foundation Trust hospitals between 2005 and 2009. The report described the inexcusable suffering of many patients within the Trust and highlighted a culture of concealment and self-protection (Francis 2013). Although the investigation was focused on one hospital, it revealed failures throughout the Trust, particularly regarding the systems that were supposed to monitor safe practice to ensure that all clients were treated with dignity and compassion – in accordance with significant government legislation, and organisational, departmental and professional/regulatory policies. The report highlighted several essential findings, including a lack of basic care in many of the wards and departments, with some distressing personal accounts of appalling neglect. Some healthcare practitioners were reported to have treated clients and their families with a lack of kindness, indifference and in some cases cruelty. Significantly, there was evidence of self-protection amongst colleagues, with team members not speaking out openly and truthfully about cases of neglect and poor care.

As far back as 2001, the concept of 'whistleblowing' (when an individual exposes misconduct, abuse, dishonesty or illegal activity within a healthcare setting) was central to the Kennedy Report (*The Report of the Public Inquiry into children's heart surgery at the Bristol Royal Infirmary 1984–1995*). Since 2001, there have been frequent media reports of whistleblowers having to face reprisals, often at the hands of the individual, organisation or group they have accused of malpractice.

In view of all this, many questions have been raised about the legitimacy of whistleblowing, the moral responsibility of whistleblowing, and how whistleblowing can be encouraged within institutions. Yet a culture of silence and fear remained a central theme when the Francis Report was published in 2013. In some cases, healthcare staff were said to be aware of the poor care but so institutionalised that it did not register. Alternatively, some of them felt too frightened to raise or pursue concerns. In other words, staff did not raise the alarm because they were probably frightened of reprisals such as losing their jobs. Considering the interval between the Kennedy Report in 2001 and the Francis Report in 2013, one has to question what, if any, improvement occurred in the 12 years between the two inquiries.

Pause and reflect

Reflect on your own workplace or a recent placement and record any incidents where you feel that something should have been said, or was said, about falling standards of care.

- What was the outcome?
- Did colleagues feel supported?
- Were any actions agreed? If not, why not?
- How did this make you feel?

The Francis Report highlighted the mental, physical, emotional and spiritual impact of falling standards and unprofessional practices when it described the extreme and inexcusable suffering of some of the most vulnerable patients (Francis 2013). The Mid Staffordshire NHS Foundation Trust public inquiry publicised failures of nursing performance and conduct that cumulatively started to undermine public confidence in all healthcare professionals. The report showed that the system as a whole had failed in its most essential duty – to protect patients from unacceptable risks of harm. It went on to describe unacceptable, and in some cases, inhumane treatment.

Thanks to the Francis Report, we now appear to have a more open and transparent healthcare service, with more emphasis on the needs of clients. It is likely that professional practice can and will be improved by means of education and training. However, this remains to be seen, as we continue to witness media coverage of major incidents of unprofessional practice and resulting prosecution from across the UK. The Nursing and Midwifery Council (2013) responded to the Francis Report by calling for better measures to ensure the quality of clinical practice, including tighter regulation. However, as Crossley *et al.* (2002) highlighted, effective professional regulation depends on effective assessment.

Although it is over ten years old, the *National service framework: older people* (DH 2001) still has a big influence on quality standards for health and social care for older adults. Its aim was to provide a clear political platform to help older people stay healthy, active and independent for as long as possible. It provided a framework to ensure that older people would be treated fairly and with respect and dignity, and that measures would be put in place to prevent unnecessary hospital admission and to give support for early discharge. It also aimed to reduce long-term illness by providing specific specialist care and to promote healthy lifestyles and independence for older people.

Nevertheless, over a decade later, concern is still being expressed as to how we can maintain dignity in care for older people. Older people are often negatively perceived and treated, and frequently have minimal influence on decisions affecting their own care, partly due to poor communication. Negative stereotypical images of older people, based on ageist assumptions, pervade our society. Older people are frequently seen as 'a burden', putting pressure on financial resources, and considered non-productive in terms of generating income and therefore less deserving. Yet it is quite possible to see ageing in a very different light – as creative rather than limiting (see Chapter 6).

The 2000 Race Relations Act and the 1998 Human Rights Act are two more key pieces of legislation. These laws emphasise the duty of organisations to treat all citizens fairly, irrespective of their background, colour, religion or personal situation. Concerns have been highlighted in the Healthcare Commission's work on race equality, as well as the response to the Joint Health Select Committee on the Human Rights of Older People in Healthcare (2007). As a result, the *Healthcare Commission Annual Report* (2007) focused on dignity as a key theme, and made a commitment to undertake targeted inspection to assess the extent to which NHS trusts are meeting standards relating to dignity in care for hospital inpatients. Through in-depth inspection of specific trusts that appear to be under-performing, and identifying and disseminating examples of good practice by benchmarking key aspects of this legislation, the Healthcare Commission aims to promote improved standards of care.

Finally, the 1998 Human Rights Act (HRA) has become one of the main drivers in safeguarding vulnerable adults in the UK. Faulkner and Sweeney (2011) see the main purpose of this act as enforcing the rights of individuals, whilst also encouraging public organisations to take responsibility for improving standards of practice. The HRA underpins the Safeguarding Adults' Policy and has direct relevance to abuse and malpractice in healthcare and social care by enshrining:

- The right to life
- The right not to be tortured or treated in an inhuman or degrading way
- The right to liberty
- The right to respect for private and family life, home and correspondence.

Again, despite such clear legislation having been passed so long ago, there have been many cases of serious abuse of vulnerable people reported within health and social care services in the UK. The HRA also stresses the importance of raising awareness and clarifying the specific responsibilities and roles of professional staff in order to protect vulnerable adults. Pritchard (2009, p. 125) states that 'adults who lack decision-making capacity are the most vulnerable in society'.

In order to safeguard clients protected by the 2005 Mental Capacity Act, the Deprivation of Liberty Safeguards came into effect in 2009. This act made registered UK hospitals and care homes responsible for seeking consent from health authorities or health boards as a priority before depriving someone with a mental health disorder of their liberty (DH 2012). Clearly, the Deprivation of Liberty Safeguards plays a significant role in protecting the human rights of individuals who are vulnerable. However, there appears to be some confusion about these measures and irregular national implementation of them. Financial challenges, fear of investigation, and inconsistencies in the management and education of professionals have all been blamed for problems in implementing the safeguards.

Understanding compassion and dignity

Britain has a diverse population and every individual's needs are influenced by a wide range of factors, including their cultural background, values and religious and spiritual beliefs. Most people would agree that compassion and dignity are complex concepts to define and are open to interpretation, based on cultural differences, individual beliefs, media perceptions and personal experience. Currently, there is no agreed standard working definition of dignity. The Oxford Dictionary describes dignity as 'the state or quality of being worthy of respect'. Meanwhile, Nordenfelt (2012) describes human dignity as a complex multi-faceted concept, with four distinct aspects: universal human value; dignity as merit; dignity as moral stature; and dignity of personal identity, including sense of self and sense of social recognition. You would have thought that there would be some common agreement on qualities we would expect of carers such as nurses, doctors or therapists. These might include: the ability to listen to clients and make them feel included; respect for clients and sensitivity about how to address them; being polite to clients, offering them choices and making them feel valued. But in some cases none of these qualities are apparent.

In 2012, NHS England set out core values in the form of the 6Cs – Care, Compassion, Competence, Communication, Courage and Commitment. These values are becoming further embedded across healthcare, as they are directly relevant to all healthcare workers, including doctors, nurses, allied health professionals and social workers (NHS Executive 2012). It is important to empower healthcare workers across the UK to embrace the 6Cs, in order to ensure that they take an approach to care that is motivated by compassion. So what is compassion in practice?

Compassion can mean many things. Some people view compassion in a similar light to having a religious or vocational calling, whilst others simply see it as having a truly caring approach to healthcare practice. It is certainly a word that has connotations of empathy, kindness, care, warmth and dignity. When we are vulnerable and suffering, we seek it in ourselves and others. The word 'compassion' has appeared in many recent national reports and inquiries, and it is clear that enormous damage and hurt can ensue when compassion is not present.

Hornett (2012) describes systems within nursing in which a combination of action research and appreciative inquiry resulted in the development of processes to support the delivery of compassionate care in practice. These systems have involved nursing in 28 specialisms, ranging from mental health to maternity processes. They included the concepts of caring conversations, flexible person-centred risk-taking, valuing and transparency, and creating an environment in which staff, clients and families could actively influence and participate in the way healthcare was practised.

Dignity is about acknowledging the innate value in every individual, especially when they are feeling vulnerable and dependent on others for aspects of their care. Compassion is the close twin of dignity – in the sense that a compassionate healthcare professional empathises with their clients and yet keeps an element of detachment in order to act efficiently to relieve suffering.

Pause and reflect

- What do the words 'compassion' and 'dignity' mean to you personally?
- Try to formulate working definitions of these terms, and think about the characteristics which demonstrate that someone is compassionate and dignified.
- In a health- or social care environment, how could you show a client that you are compassionate and that you respect their dignity?

We use the term 'person-centred care', rather than 'client-centred care', in order to emphasise the importance of seeing the whole person – beyond the constraints of their diagnosis or their particular situation. In recent years, this message has been strongly conveyed by the 'hello my name is' social media campaign. This was initiated by Dr Kate Granger, a terminally ill hospital consultant who became frustrated with the number of healthcare staff who failed to introduce themselves to her when she was an inpatient with post-operative sepsis. In essence she views the system as inhumane and unable to see the whole person. And, in her experience, she was told what to do, rather than being empowered to make choices herself.

Person-centred care is often talked about, but is it a reality for our clients? In a world where litigation is increasingly common, do we dare to put clients at the very heart of all key decisions pertaining to their care? Being treated as an individual, and having your personal needs considered and met, are undoubtedly key aspects of dignity in practice. Clients have expectations regarding attention and personal care, effective communication, the provision of a good healthy diet and adequate privacy. Yet older people, in particular, often find that their treatment is less than satisfactory in terms of dignity. Although they may find it hard to define the concept of dignity, older people and their carers find it easy to describe situations where their dignity has been compromised or their care has not been respectful or compassionate.

Sadly, the truth is that many vulnerable people (especially older adults) are ill-treated in our care system. Abuse in care settings is not a new phenomenon, and vulnerable people have the same human right as anyone – to demand good-quality care, free of exploitation and mental or physical abuse. For example, Tadd and Bayer (2006) believe that dignity is a complex concept, subject to a range of different interpretations. The Royal College of Nursing (2008) emphasises the core nursing values of respect and autonomy, rather than care delivery, when defining dignity. The RCN makes it clear that dignity is essentially concerned with how individuals feel, think and behave, in relation to their own sense of worth and that of others. The worth element is paramount. To treat someone with dignity is to treat them as being of worth, in a way that respects them as valued individuals within society.

In a study of clients' and carers' perceptions of dignity, Cairns *et al.* (2013) found that older people and their relatives focused on the importance of satisfactory physical care when describing what dignity meant to them. They also emphasised the importance of the more relational aspects of care delivery, which are often overlooked, ignored or undervalued. The Social Care Institute for Excellence (2010) states that the relational aspects of a dignified and caring attitude are at the heart of a person-centred approach to care. This person-centred approach means enabling clients to maintain the maximum possible degree of independence, choice and control over their own lives. It also requires care workers to give clients the same level of respect they would want for themselves or their own loved ones.

Calnan *et al.* (2006) reported that older people saw respect, privacy, good communication, and being treated in a person-centred way as important aspects of dignified care. Again, the majority of participants in the study emphasised basic physical aspects of care (such as eating, nutrition, personal hygiene and toileting) as central to them feeling as if professionals were treating them with dignity and compassion. Cairns *et al.* (2013) states that one in five hospitals inspected by the Care Quality Commission in 2011 showed basic failings on dignity and nutrition.

Competence to practice

Professional competence remains central to all aspects of professional regulation and is seen as a minimum requirement to practice. But what do we understand by the word 'competent', and – more importantly – how do we judge incompetence? Some may see incompetence as not being sufficiently qualified or not being able to perform a particular task or showing a lack of informed knowledge and skill. An incompetent care worker may carry out unsafe, harmful, unscrupulous and, as we have seen in the Francis Report (2013), undignified and uncompassionate, and even unlawful, actions. Some of the problems and challenges of performance and conduct are encapsulated in the way we define these terms.

Pause and reflect

Consider your own professional competence.

- Are your qualifications and experience up to date and appropriate for your job as a healthcare worker?
- What advice would you give your own professional body about the competencies needed to carry out your role safely and to a high standard?

Many would argue that the concept of incompetence has received little attention in the caring professions' literature. This may be partly due to the oft-mentioned norm of non-criticism, which has historically almost amounted to a tolerance of incompetence.

However, with an increasing focus on clinical governance tools (including professional regulation, clinical audits and more transparent complaints procedures), this has started to change. The 'silence' has been further broken by the general public's greater confidence in expressing their concerns and demanding accountability and responsibility from healthcare practitioners.

Empathy

Empathy is a word that is often used and discussed in the caring environment. It is suggested that through the care worker's empathic sharing, the feelings and emotions of the client, their current state, situation and thinking can be identified. This allows the care worker to be more appreciative and to address major issues of immediate concern to the client. Having said this, the use of the word empathy has many challenges. Although definitions of the word vary, the term essentially refers to being able to 'stand in the client's shoes' as a way of sharing their feelings and as a means of coming to a direct appreciation of their situation – at a time when they are often at their most vulnerable. 'Empathy' is often contrasted with the term 'sympathy', which is more about identifying with the client's feelings, rather than their whole situation.

To find the optimum practical, emotional and behavioural approach to caring, practitioners may need to consider adopting an alternative to empathy. Some may prefer the use of the word 'caring' on its own, as it perhaps better expresses both an emotional reaction to the client and the expression of that empathic response in everyday practice. In a healthcare context, true caring involves astute observation, accurate assessment, focused listening (and hearing), and responsive, appreciative questioning. When caring is carried out in this way, in harmony with the needs of the client, professional intervention is stripped of any unhelpful assumptions about what the client may or may not be experiencing.

All care professionals should have the ability to read cues in clients' word choices, posture, actions and gestures. Tuning in to these from a place of genuine attention, in a non-threatening, open-hearted and empathic way, gives a clear message that we care. In the context of compassion and dignity, empathy can be seen as a form of emotional engagement that is beneficial to the quality of client care. However, when we look at empathy in this way, the very word may lead to mistaken assumptions and an absence of corrective curiosity. For example, some care workers may think that they understand what the client is experiencing. They may listen to the client but not actually validate and respond to their needs. Thus, excessively empathic care workers do not empower the client to act, and may fail to provide high-quality, person-centred, compassionate and dignified care. When the care worker empowers the client to make their own choices, they find the bridge between empathy and compassion. A truly compassionate care worker is motivated to act in order to alleviate or end the suffering of the client. This will be explored and developed more fully in Chapters 6, 7 and 8.

Conclusion

In the context of decreasing financial resources, there is little doubt that healthcare workers and leaders are struggling to meet the increasing needs and expectations of clients, patients and carers. Healthcare professionals have a responsibility to guarantee patient safety, and research across many countries clearly shows that they are committed to this. In particular, nurses play a key role in delivering high-quality, safe, compassionate and dignified care in practice (Ross 2011, Ball *et al.* 2013, Kirwan *et al.* 2013, You *et al.* 2013). With demands for professionals and support workers to do more with less, in addition to societal changes, changing values, work ethics and stress, there are strong indicators that our precious human resources are burning out. Often it appears that authentic care and compassion are not prevalent in some areas of healthcare. At different times and under different circumstances, the same person may be capable of caring or not caring, being compassionate or not. Sustaining good care and best practice depends on us managing ourselves in such a way that work pressures trigger resilient and conscious caring, rather than blind, careless reaction.

There appears to be a disconnect between healthcare professionals' and clients' ideas of what is truly meant by compassion and dignity. Various reports and inquiries have indicated that some professionals do not attribute enough importance to caring, and what it means to be cared for. Care policies appear to be interpreted differently by different professional groups. According to Cairns *et al.* (2013), there is some evidence that these policies are being interpreted 'as an approach towards care' and not being applied to direct care provision. This limited interpretation may help to explain society's concern about the continued neglect of older people, particularly in acute settings. It is therefore crucial that all care personnel (whether they are support workers, policy makers, cleaners, porters, managers, directors, chief executives, medical doctors, allied health professionals, healthcare students or social workers) realise that they have an equal duty to provide conscious, respectful, compassionate and dignified care.

In this chapter, we have examined the main policy influences, and key aspects of compassion and dignity. We have also touched on levels of competence and behaviours associated with professionalism in care. In the next chapter, we will explore what is expected of a professional care worker in practice or a healthcare student on placement, identifying what professionalism means, and how lapses can be identified in practice.

Chapter 2

Professionalism – on becoming a professional

Introduction

This chapter looks critically at what society expects of professional healthcare practitioners, students and all those who constitute a multi-disciplinary team. It will help to identify what professionalism means, and how lapses can be identified in practice. Although the literature acknowledges the desirability of addressing and improving professionalism, the concept of 'professionalism' is not generally well-defined, conceptually or methodologically (HCPC 2014).

This chapter should be of equal relevance for healthcare students and qualified and non-qualified professionals and support practitioners. Irrespective of professional qualifications, background or status, all healthcare workers need a solid understanding of what it means to care. According to the *Nursing Times* (2013), the concept of professionalism is the best regulator of health- and social care. Nevertheless, on reading the Francis Report (2013), no professional practitioner could fail to be concerned about the dreadful and unnecessary suffering of patients in a place the public would have regarded as safe and with professionals they thought they could trust. The Francis Report gave a strong message that those responsible for recruitment, retention and training of nurses must ensure high quality in registered nurses – in terms of their ethics as well as what they do in practice.

Professionalism, with its associated standards and values at all levels in the workplace, lies at the heart of the matter. All qualified healthcare professionals work to a professional code, with competencies and standards of conduct, performance and ethics that should be applied to themselves and any other workers they may be regulating. Leaders and managers need to know that any professional healthcare worker they employ will follow the relevant professional code and standards, and action needs to be taken if they fail to do so. If, as happened with the whistleblowing attempts made by some Mid Staffordshire

Trust nurses, professionalism is not respected internally by management, and failings are not picked up externally, there is potentially a serious gap in respective professional frameworks (*Nursing Times* 2013), and the consequences can be as appalling as those highlighted in the Francis Report.

Healthcare practitioners and their education should not stand still, nor should the expectations of the society they serve. Individual professional practice, knowledge, behaviour and skill are often seen as the main determiners of good or bad care/practice – but is this still the case? Healthcare practitioners often have a 'professional-centric' view of the world. However we must not allow professional elitism to limit what is essential to healthcare, which is cross-functional collaboration and multi-disciplinary team working, where extended scope practice is now actively promoted. In addition, the organisations that healthcare practitioners work for, and the professional associations they belong to, have historically upheld what Ovretveit, Mathias and Thompson (1997) saw as 'the myth of the omnipotence of the individual practitioner'.

Most of us don't think about healthcare services, or the people who work in them, until we have to – either because we ourselves or one of our loved ones needs medical treatment or social care. People who work in care are drawn from a broad cross-section of the working population and the whole system depends on having a variety of highly qualified, well-trained professionals working alongside dedicated and committed support personnel. While it would be unrealistic to claim that we can guarantee safe, competent, compassionate and honourable practice by all professionals all the time, members of the public have a right to expect the most rigorous enforcement of procedures and protocols aiming to fulfil this aspiration. This chapter is intended to offer a better understanding of the many complex factors that influence professional practice.

Factors influencing professionalism

As discussed in Chapter 1, although there appear to have been significant developments in policies and legislation to ensure competency and professionalism, the media have still exposed cases of serious abuse, bad care and neglect. For instance, an independent inquiry into the deaths of many elderly patients, given what was termed 'life shortening' powerful painkillers, addressed the damning audit of deaths at Gosport War Memorial Hospital (Baker 2013). The audit, carried out by Professor Richard Baker who also worked on the Harold Shipman inquiry, found evidence of highly unprofessional practice, with morphine and other strong sedatives being routinely prescribed for elderly patients even when they were not in pain. The inquiry found that the routine use of such drugs had in essence shortened the lives of some individuals who might otherwise have been discharged from hospital alive. Yet the Baker Report was suppressed by the government for several years. How can we, moving forward, ensure that such information is not hidden or denied on political grounds?

On reading both the Baker and Francis reports, it is clear that all members of the workforce, in all settings and sectors, have an essential role to play in learning lessons from scandals that have been exposed. Although the recommendations in these reports are limited to England, they raise important issues of professionalism for all services in Wales, Scotland and Northern Ireland (and should, of course, be of interest to all international colleagues). Whilst the Francis investigation was focused on one particular NHS Foundation Trust, it showed that there was a failure throughout the health and social care systems and by a wide range of professional groups who were supposed to monitor safe practice to ensure that patients were treated with dignity and care, in accordance with government legislation and departmental policies.

The publication of the Francis Report has arguably gone some way towards changing what is generally understood as professionalism in care, and has raised awareness of what happens when standards fall as a result of unprofessional practice. Indeed, its findings have played a key role in changing expectations and have been a significant influence on our understanding of what is expected of a healthcare professional. The Francis Report has also given society as a whole the confidence to question and challenge sub-standard care and unprofessional practices, and bring professional accountability to the forefront of regulations.

Furthermore, the Francis Report has helped organisations and policy makers to raise and maintain standards, as well as highlighting each individual healthcare practitioner's accountability, and their responsibility to continually develop their own professional skills, knowledge and attitude – in other words, the concept of life-long learning and continuing professional development (CPD).

The 290 recommendations made in the Francis Report emphasise the accountability required of all care practitioners. Some of the key recommendations continue to have a significant influence in areas such as adult safeguarding policy. These include the following points:

- Accountability for implementation of the recommendations, which requires all persons caring for service-users to be dedicated in implementing a safer and compassionate service, whilst remaining open and transparent.
- A putting of the patient first –the NHS must put the patient first in everything it does. Within available resources, they must receive effective services from caring, compassionate and committed staff, working within a common culture, and they must be protected from avoidable harm and any deprivation of their basic rights.

- Effective complaints handling – Patients raising concerns about their care are entitled to: have the matter dealt with as a complaint unless they do not wish it; identification of their expectations; prompt and thorough processing; sensitive, responsive and accurate communication; effective and implemented learning; and proper and effective communication of the complaint to those responsible for providing the care.

  (Francis 2013, pp. 85–115)

The report does not focus on any single key professional group, and in fact has significant implications for all, as the policy requires everyone to take ownership of their own practice in ensuring the dignity, safety and respect of all clients. It goes further by recommending that all healthcare practitioners put the patient first. But how can this be achieved? What professional influences do we need to consider in order to ensure that such ownership and accountability become ingrained in healthcare practice and education, at both undergraduate and postgraduate level, so that current and future healthcare practitioners are truly 'professional in their caring'? To achieve this, we believe that caring must be seen as a vital opportunity, rather than simply a challenge. Seeing difficult situations merely as problems may not be a constructive way forward.

Professional practice

People hear the word 'professional' but do they really understand the concept of professionalism or the character traits required to be a true professional? Health- and social care practitioners like to be described as 'professional', despite the fact that professions and their members are often regarded with a certain amount of suspicion and mistrust. But do we understand terms such as professional, professionalism or professionalisation? And how do we uphold the values and beliefs commonly associated with professional practice in healthcare? When describing a professional, we may say that they:

- Have specialist knowledge
- Have core knowledge
- Strive to offer a high-quality service
- Achieve and maintain high standards
- Follow ethical practices
- Work to a set of agreed minimum standards
- Have achieved a certain level of competence
- Are a specialist
- Have achieved personal mastery.

To be involved in a profession, or to benefit from professional intervention, involves engaging with that particular profession's values. These values are expressed in oaths, codes of practice, mission statements, charters and all sorts of different individual and occupational behaviours. Yet, whilst such values are often discussed, they are seldom examined or critically understood.

In the same way, terms like 'profession' and 'professional' can be understood in various ways by people within and outside an organisation. Before considering the true meaning of these terms, it may be helpful to pause and reflect on your own use of the noun 'profession', the noun and adjective 'professional' and the adverb 'professionally'.

Pause and reflect

- How do you use the term 'profession' and 'professional' and for what purpose?
- How would you describe professional practice in care?
- What constitutes being a professional and belonging to a professional body?

Professions and the people who belong to them are continually changing, as are society's expectations. For example, behaviour and conduct that was acceptable two decades ago may now be unacceptable. Consequently, each profession needs to keep re-evaluating what constitutes integrated competence as the world changes around them. Thus, an allied health professional or nurse who fails to scrutinise another's performance could find themselves being reported to the Health and Care Professions Council (HCPC) or the Nursing and Midwifery Council (NMC).

Pause and reflect

- Have there been incidents in your professional life when you've questioned a colleague's actions, behaviour or attitude towards someone?
- If so, what would you do if it happened now? And how would you go about expressing your concerns?
- Would you think of commenting on a colleague's professionalism if you witnessed exceptional or exemplary care?

Individuals, groups and communities deal with each other and the outside world on the basis of shared values, beliefs and assumptions, which make up our culture. This culture is reflected in our behaviour and language, the groups we belong to, and the very nature of our society. In this context, it is complex and challenging to agree on a standard definition of professionalism.

Modern society is increasingly challenging professionals to justify their professional actions, behaviours, decisions, judgements, roles and level of knowledge and skill. Evidence-based practice, clinical guidelines, certain initiatives and advances in treatment all come into play to assist the professional in describing and explaining their own roles and actions. In addition, professional values are closely connected to deeply held convictions about the rights of those served and the obligations of the individual practitioner (Roberts 2005). A value often has a moral, ethical, or philosophical basis concerning what is considered right, good, just or desirable. Thus, values are viewed as a means of unifying the profession, providing a unique professional identity, and promoting coherent, safe practice.

Both individuals and employing organisations need to make a commitment to continuing professional development (CPD) so that professionals keep up to date with developments in their discipline and hence offer clients the best possible care. 'Professional development' refers to the activities that care workers undertake to ensure that they provide an ever higher quality of service and strive for the highest level of attainment and/or responsibility in their work area. 'Personal development' activities refer to all other (not strictly professional development) activities, such as training intended to equip carers with skills or experience that can be beneficial to their practice and area of work, but not directly linked to it (Murray & Simpson 2000). CPD is often linked with discussions about the government's quality and clinical governance agenda. All professional and regulatory bodies have incorporated personal and organisational accountability, and responsibility for maintaining CPD, for many years.

Impact of unprofessional practice

Cases referred to professional regulators are often linked to a wide range of attitudes and behaviours, and may not necessarily involve lack of technical ability. When professionalism is questioned or malpractice is observed, people frequently complain about not being cared for in the manner they expected to be cared for by the people they placed their trust in, at a time when they were at their most vulnerable. When accessing any service (public or private), we all run the risk of encountering unprofessional attitudes and behaviours that may lead us to question the quality of care within that service. In healthcare, some unprofessional behaviour and practice has, as we know, resulted in harm, mistreatment, abuse and even death.

The Department of Health (2000a, p. 9), defines abuse as 'a violation of an individual's human and civil rights by any other person or persons'. History has shown that the most vulnerable groups, such as older adults and young children, are particularly prone to such abuse and mistreatment. The Department of Health also describes a vulnerable adult as an individual 'who is or may be in need of community care services by reason of mental or other disability, age or illness and who is or may be unable to take care of him or herself, or unable to protect him or herself against significant harm or exploitation' (DH 2000b, p. 9).

Currently, the Human Rights Act (HRA 1998) remains the main driver in developing provision for safeguarding vulnerable adults within Europe, as it ensures that the law enforces the rights of all individuals, whilst encouraging public organisations to keep improving their standards of practice. The HRA underpins health and social care policies relating to safeguarding and is particularly relevant in areas such as the right to life, the right not to be tortured or treated in an inhuman or degrading way, the right to liberty and the right to respect for private and family life, home and correspondence. These rights need to be borne in mind because sadly some serious inquiry reports into failing health and social care services have shown them being ignored and overlooked.

Professional boundaries and inter-professional working

The inward-looking, elitist and inflexible behaviour of some professional groups creates a 'silo' mentality, whereby each organisation jealously guards its own information and refuses to share it with other organisations involved in the care of a particular individual or group. References to these 'elitist' profession-specific teams, who do not work effectively and in partnership with other care services, have appeared in the literature and within the inquiries mentioned. For example, there have been several historical examples of a lack of collaboration and cooperative working when carrying out client assessment.

In view of these problems, the concept of inter-professional, multi-disciplinary and multi-agency team working has become a central component in health and social care, and a more integrated and unified approach is now being taken to assessment. In this way, innovative ideas and practices can be modelled, shared and adopted by a wide range of colleagues and professionals, thus enhancing client care. Ross and McSherry (2010, p. 162) argue that some practices are not transferrable, as, for example, 'some tools used in social work or family therapy will include strategies that may not be suitable for nurses admitting patients onto acute hospital wards'. Yet, despite the varying contexts, evidence is emerging to show that different professional groups and individual practitioners, when working in partnership, can construct, utilise and share a wide variety of assessment strategies.

The Francis Report (2013) emphasises the importance of such shared strategies, in addition to staff teamwork and engagement with clients and carers, as important ways to achieve the implementation of a collaborative culture. Professional disengagement within teams was identified as a serious flaw in developments at the Mid Staffordshire Foundation Trust. The report also highlighted lack of accountability and increased passivity about difficult personnel issues within teams, with consultants not being at the forefront of promoting change.

Overall, the report suggests that a more rigorous inter-professional, multi-agency approach is required to provide a safe system for clients. Such cross-boundary collaboration would strengthen the sense of collective responsibility and help ensure that good-quality care is delivered at every level, by all professionals and support workers. Teams should aim to provide a service in which the boundaries between primary healthcare, secondary healthcare, social care and the voluntary sector do not form barriers, seen from the perspective of the client. In policy terms, multi-agency, cross-boundary team working is now the preferred method of overcoming challenges. This approach also requires an increasing commitment on the part of universities to advocate and validate undergraduate inter-professional learning and education opportunities for the medical, health and social care workers of the future.

There is a clear need to collaborate across service and professional boundaries in order to tackle perceived inequalities in service delivery. Yet there are still some professional and organisational barriers that can inhibit effective high-quality care services. An important aspect of being professional is to address such barriers so as to achieve greater integration across the primary care/local authority divide. Allied health professionals and nurses now take a more prominent role and this has helped further the objectives of creating better-integrated services and closer, more respectful inter-professional working.

In the past decade, overcoming professional boundaries has become one of the key goals in health and social service provision. However, to some, the speed of change in implementing fully integrated services appears far too slow. Nevertheless, the impact of change has been experienced by all health and social care professionals, especially in the development of partnership initiatives involving nurses and allied health professionals. This move towards cross-boundary working, both between and within professions, has pushed professional relationships to new heights (Roberts 2005). Boundaries between agencies and professionals often come into being through differences in organisational structures and values (Stantham 2000), and through professional elitist beliefs.

Pause and reflect

- Are you operating within your chosen professional role?
- Are you referring clients on to other professionals if these clients need areas of competence that you lack?
- Reflect on how you reconcile the personal and professional aspects of your relationship with each client.
- Which code of ethics and professional practices do you subscribe to?

- Reflect on your own views of some other professionals within your team. If any of these views are preconceived, biased, negative or prejudiced, how can you go about changing them in yourself and others?

Enhancing professionalism – a more appreciative approach

Every healthcare professional will benefit from having excellent problem-solving skills, as we all encounter challenges that need to be overcome on a daily basis. Some of these challenges are obviously more complex and difficult than others but it is clear that problem-solving and decision-making are key skills for any healthcare professional and support worker. In this context, problem-solving often involves informed decision-making as an important aspect of managing oneself and others. Later on, in Chapter 4, we consider the relevance of appreciative inquiry (AI), used alongside the problem-solving process. The problem-solving cycle allows professionals to identify their clients' strengths and weaknesses but AI goes further, by empowering professionals to use an enhanced and adapted model of problem-solving with individual clients. This approach creates and sustains the energy needed to realise a more positively envisioned future.

AI is a high-engagement strengths-based process, through which people collaboratively identify a positive core in all that they do and say. It is an approach to thinking and learning that is based on affirmative action and visions of the possible, rather than finding what is wrong and looking for difficulties (Cooperrider & Whitney 2005). We argue that the positive strengths of AI naturally balance the limitations of a more problem-solving approach (Machon & Roberts 2010). This is an exciting new application of AI in a healthcare context, which we believe will have an affirmative impact on professionalism and person-centred care, thus furthering the compassionate and dignified care agenda. The ultimate aim is to create a new foundation for enabling positive, transformative change in the way we care. Problem-solving is discussed in Chapter 3, and AI is discussed in more detail in Chapter 4.

Change is the essence

Leaders who guide the destinies of healthcare organisations are now facing an unprecedented set of demands and dilemmas. Clients, families and healthcare professionals have identified an urgent need for a systematic inquiry into the leadership and management of fundamental change in the NHS. Yet there is often a tension between dealing with short-term urgent pressures and addressing the strategic management of an entire healthcare organisation. Significant professional leadership and energy are required to get the balance right.

Professionalism dictates that we must have a clear vision of the desired end state of the entire system, including its core business and its ways of working. This vision must be used both to diagnose the need to change and also to manage the process of change, thus acting as a force to integrate the many disparate changes that must be made. Above all, there must be an intergrated plan for making the changes, and all healthcare professionals and agencies must sign up to it.

Pause and reflect

Consider how you personally may be able to influence this agenda.

- What qualities do you have that could enable you to be part of this fundamental change?
- What is your personal and professional strategy to achieve excellence in practice?

Reflect on your workplace and/or learning environment and consider what needs to change in order to realise this affirmative agenda.

- What are your own continuing professional development needs and how will fulfilling them enhance your professionalism?

Conclusion

The first step towards this fundamental change must be to make a conscious decision to move to an affirmative and professional practice and learning mode, in which both learning and actions are equally valued and where individual and collective excellence in care is celebrated. This affirmative approach is an essential precondition for managing fundamental change in healthcare. Furthermore, all professionals, practitioners, manager leaders and lobbyists have to commit to investing significant time and energy in developing this inspirational and affirmative vision. To this end, we all need to behave in ways that are congruent with this vision of mindful, conscious, compassionate, dignified, professionally led care.

Chapter 3

Problem-solving in healthcare

Introduction

This chapter will look at the traditional problem-solving approach that is often applied in healthcare systems. We will also examine the way pedagogical approaches, such as problem-based learning (PBL), continue to influence professional practice and healthcare education. We introduce the reader to the 'analytical eye', the first of the three lenses in our model of practice, which will be examined in greater detail in Chapter 6. In this chapter, we analyse some of the challenges faced by healthcare workers and students, and investigate how the problem-solving approach can limit our approach and may often make us overlook the interactive and relational aspects of care.

This chapter will replicate a problem-solving approach as applied in practice. It will also replicate PBL as a pedagogical approach applied to healthcare education.
In essence, both follow the same path:

In practice: assess – plan – intervene – evaluate

In PBL: identify what needs to be learned – research – plan – intervene – evaluate.

The problem-solving cycle

When we truly care for another person, we are not using that person to satisfy our own needs; and we are doing more than just wishing them well, or liking, comforting, or merely being interested in what happens to them. As Mayeroff (1971) argued, we are helping clients to grow, to progress in some way, to get better. Caring is a way of relating to someone that involves development. This remains consistent throughout the entire process of care, from initial arrival and assessment to identification of the problem, thoughtful intervention and evaluation, discharge and beyond. When we offer professional services, and attend to another person in a manner based on unconditional caring, we need to be aware of our own values and beliefs and how these may affect our professional practice.

This is key to the whole healthcare intervention process but it is particularly important when assessing a client's needs.

The problem-solving process often follows the healthcare intervention 'assess – plan – intervene – evaluate' cycle, as described by Polglase and Tresender (2012, pp. 53–107).

Assessment

The assessment is used to gather a broad baseline of information about a client in order to plan intervention. Such a gathering of intelligence should equip the carer with an accurate perspective on both the challenges and the opportunities facing the client. Yet assessment commonly focuses on 'what is wrong', 'what are the main problems and/or challenges' and 'what the individual is unable to achieve'. In essence, assessment is most commonly deficit-based.

Planning

Planning involves using assessment information to formulate an intervention plan. Based on the information gathered, the practitioner works with the multi-disciplinary team to decide on what further assessments are needed in order to formulate a clear intervention strategy. Teams agree on how best to progress and plan specific therapeutic, medical or nursing strategies.

Intervention

When making professional interventions, the plan is effectively implemented. Care workers combine their individual and collective specialist knowledge and skill to achieve what is assessed to be the very best outcome for the client.

Evaluation

Finally, the overall cycle is evaluated to determine whether the problem has been solved. This stage involves critical analysis and reflection against an outcome measure. Creek (2010, p. 25) defines evaluation as 'the process of obtaining, interpreting and appraising information in order to prioritise problems and needs, to plan and modify interventions and judge their worth'.

In focusing on the problem, the above intervention cycle mirrors a process that a significant number of professionals would traditionally follow in healthcare settings. The main requirement is to identify the significant presenting challenges faced by clients. Individuals may arrive at a healthcare setting with a wide range of problems, ranging from minor cuts and bruises to complex and life-threatening illnesses. A straightforward problem is one for which a full, reasonable, logical, conclusive solution can be found. For instance, there is no doubt about whether a femur is fractured because an X-ray can prove it to be so. The answer to this problem (the treatment required) remains the same and the context does not necessarily matter. Nevertheless, it must be remembered that the fractured femur is only the diagnosis; there is also a real human being who has to attempt to live an active and meaningful life while the injury heals.

Such problems can be 'fixed'. They are consistent and quantitative and can be analytically assessed according to the pure medical model. But some presenting problems have to be addressed in a less than conclusive fashion. In fact, a greater proportion of these problems are qualitative and inhabit a social (rather than medical) model of care. A caring approach is therefore commonly seen to be more qualitative – and, in our terms, less analytical and more appreciative.

Orem, Binkert and Clancy (2007) remind us of how context matters. For instance, when healthcare workers only focus on the client's problems and needs, they often forget to recognise and evaluate what the client achieved before the illness or disability, and what they have achieved since. We also need to bear in mind the notion of 'can do', and celebrate success and achievements, irrespective of disability or diagnosis.

Healthcare workers, by default, tend to ask clients more negative than affirmative questions. Polglase and Tresender (2012, p. 53) view assessment as the initial phase in which practitioners gather 'information about the service user in order to plan intervention collaboratively with them'. This process crucially focuses on client need, and may limit the care worker's ability to gain a broader understanding of the individual. They are likely to ask the client questions such as:

- What can't you do?
- What are your main problems and challenges?
- What skills have you lost due to your disability?
- What activities of daily living can't you independently complete?
- What occupations or activities are compromised?

In order to gather as much information as possible about the client, and truly understand their suffering and the challenges they face, it is crucial to identify the core presenting problem as seen by the client and as seen by the care worker. However, there are significant benefits in also looking beyond the challenges to see the opportunities – the areas where the client remains independently in charge, the 'can do' scenarios. By only focusing on the problem, healthcare professionals and students alike may not see the whole person, and could therefore end up not giving person-centred, compassionate and dignified care. In these circumstances, person-centred practice is in danger of being diluted and devalued, as a consequence of taking a partial, limited view of the client. To address this concern, care workers should also be willing and able to ask the client:

- What can you do?
- What have you achieved?
- What opportunities have come your way as a result of your situation?
- What basic skills can you achieve independently?
- What occupations do you still have mastery of?
- What are your aspirations?
- What do you value?
- What are your positive beliefs?
- What gives your life meaning?

Do we therefore fail the client by not being person-centred in our approach to their situation? Balancing this focus on what an individual cannot achieve (problem-solving assessment/interviewing) with an equal emphasis on what they can achieve (appreciative assessment/interviewing) offers a much more complete perspective. Appreciative interviewing is described as part of the wider appreciative inquiry (AI) process in Chapter 4, where we will explore the **appreciative eye** in detail.

We believe that making an appreciative assessment is a vital aspect of caring. This type of assessment is a new, creative and arguably central development in delivering compassionate and dignified care. Educational philosophy in current practice, as well as the education and training of the future workforce within our universities, therefore needs to embrace this vital change. A more affirmative and positive approach, such as AI, helps fulfil the aspiration to be more person-centred and can be applied proactively by both care workers and educators. Indeed, it defines the emergence of the appreciative healthcare practitioner.

Problem-based learning (PBL)

Student-centred learning appears to mirror client-centred practice (Sadlo 2004). A basic definition of PBL is provided by Boud and Feletti (1997, p. 15), which describes the process as 'an approach to structuring the curriculum which involves confronting students with problems from practice which provide a stimulus for learning'. The belief that clients should take what responsibility they can for their own health is also reflected in PBL, in that the student takes responsibility for identifying their own learning needs through self-directed learning (Biggs 2003). Rather than being prescriptive, a compassionate and caring professional should be seen as an enabler who facilitates health and well-being. In the same way, an educator needs to facilitate students' learning, rather than dictating information in a didactic manner.

There is evidence showing that a PBL-based health- and social care undergraduate programme can enhance students' approaches to studying, their perceptions of the quality of the course delivery, their concept of learning and their academic attainment (Savin-Baden & Major 2004). PBL seems to presuppose more complex conceptions of learning on the part of the students, and more student-centred conceptions of learning and teaching on the part of their tutors.

Can PBL facilitation therefore promote the development of students' conceptions of learning? And do students with a didactic idea of learning, and tutors with a tutor-centred concept of teaching, have difficulty adapting to problem-based, problem-solving curricula. In particular, problem-based curricula seem to be more effective than subject-based curricula in promoting development in conceptions of learning, thus benefiting students' capabilities as lifelong learners. It can also be argued that PBL actually presupposes more sophisticated ideas about learning on the part of the students, and this might explain why some students have difficulty adapting to it. Thus, students who approach learning as mere regurgitation of information, through exposure to a subject-based curriculum, may have considerable difficulty adapting to a problem-based curriculum.

Producing high-quality graduates (equipped with the required level of knowledge and skill as well as sound compassionate and dignified attitudes to practice) requires exposure to a variety of approaches, including: a deep approach based on understanding the meaning of the teaching materials; a surface approach based on memorising the course materials for the purposes of assessments and examinations; and, above all, plentiful opportunities to apply theory to practice through exposure to real-life situations in practice. The choice of a particular approach to studying depends on the content, the context and the demands of specific learning tasks. Changes in the design and mode of delivery of specific courses can affect the way students tackle the content. Appropriate course design, and effective facilitation of the method or nature of assessment, can therefore have a big influence on the success (or otherwise) of learning.

PBL and other teaching interventions may not be effective unless they also bring about changes in students' perceptions of themselves, and this highlights the importance of reflection and self-awareness (Lambros 2004). All healthcare students need to possess a broad and varied set of competencies as they commence academic life and work their way through to graduating and eventually entering professional practice. Reflection is defined by Roseneder, Lancee and Crowder (2004, p. 45) as 'a comparative and evaluative process of thinking'. Reflective learning encourages students to explore and understand the learning process and its impact upon them, leading to deeper learning and an enhanced learning experience.

All healthcare workers should embrace reflective learning in their quest to develop into genuine reflective practitioners, able to meet the requirements of modern-day practice whilst maximising the full potential of their education and training. Kolb's experiential learning cycle (Kolb 1984) maps learning as the experience of concrete activity, followed by reflective observation. It also outlines students' ability to reflect on and understand their own emotional experience, in order to promote their intellectual, behavioural and professional growth within the framework of emotional intelligence. When carefully applied and understood, PBL strategies can potentially enhance student learning and development by providing a systematic and methodological way to deal with problems. But is this sufficient or appropriate if it drives the students to think in a more limited and non-person-centred way?

Case study (Part 1)

In a study by Roberts (2013), the following scenario was given to three first-year PBL groups studying occupational therapy. Students were asked to reflect on a photograph showing a dishevelled young man, with long hair, cradling an old dog in the doorway of a high-street shop on a rainy day. He was holding an empty cup of coffee. He spoke to no one, just looked down.

Based purely on this visual trigger, students were asked to identify their learning needs, and what information they would require in order to best understand this scenario. No associated verbal or written prompts were given, so students had to make many assumptions.

Half the students followed the traditional PBL/problem-solving cycle. This experiment was carried out with similar groups four years in succession, and the results were consistent across all groups.

Common assumptions made by the students were:
- The individual was homeless.
- He had associated mental health problems.
- He had associated drug and alcohol problems.
- His behaviour was manipulative because he was using the dog to get money to feed his habit.
- He had poor hygiene and personal care.
- He was a societal nuisance.
- He was occupationally deprived.
- This was an example of abuse of the welfare state.

These students were taking a purely problem-solving approach, and it is noticeable that most of them saw the image as a problem to be solved. Their assessment was predominantly analytical and negative, and in some cases prejudiced. Their assumptions were largely based on stereotypes and how society tends to view homeless people in general. This shows how PBL can sometimes lead to misleading conclusions, and an alternative, more realistic, inquiry-focused approach may give a broader understanding.

The outcome of the same study with the rest of the student groups, whose learning was influenced by appreciative inquiry, will be discussed in Chapter 4.

The shortcomings of PBL

When researching the validity of PBL, McKenna and Supyk (2006) identified the challenges faced by tutors and healthcare students when over-focusing on a problem (as shown by the above example) and the need to solve problems – that is, critically evaluate and answer them. Similar concerns are highlighted in other studies by Roberts (2010), and Rubin, Kerrell and Roberts (2011), which showed that the focus on problem-solving sometimes limited students' creativity and can thus also limit the potential of person-centred practice. These researchers carried out focus groups with first-year occupational therapy students, which showed that students experienced difficulties when using the PBL approach. For instance, any outcome that fell short of a solution was seen to be a failure and resulted in increased anxiety. The study also found that students thought that using an appreciative approach, in addition to PBL, positively influenced their interactions on placements, making them more inclined to consider clients in a broader, person-centred way.

To put it another way, a rational, problem-solving approach may tend to keep students 'in their heads' and keep them out of touch 'with their hearts'. Appreciative inquiry (AI), as discussed in the next chapter, suggests that we expand our vision to accommodate what is working well. In fact, in many ways PBL and AI appear to be naturally complementary (Machon & Roberts 2010, Roberts 2013). The development of transferable skills through this new approach may therefore enhance the learning experience and clinical practice of students and the approach taken by their practice educators. This approach is more person-centred and yet, at the same time, invites us to apply technical expertise, knowledge and professional skill to practice.

Assessing student learning is one of the most powerful and affirmative roles a practice/clinical educator or nurse teacher undertakes. Assessment provides feedback for both learners and teachers. It identifies strengths, as well as areas for improvement, and can enhance motivation and personal development (Quinn & Hughes 2007). Assessment of teaching and learning is also an essential way of maintaining standards of quality and performance (Quality Assurance Agency 2007). Healthcare education now places more emphasis on the academic curriculum, and higher education institutes (HEIs) are responsible for ensuring that staff members are fit to practice, in order to protect the safety and well-being of the general public (NMC 2010). It is therefore important that student assessment include the key elements of reliability and validity, whilst also adhering to standards driven by, for example, the NMC (2010) and the Quality Assurance Agency (2007), as well as other professional regulatory bodies.

Within nursing and midwifery, for example, the NMC decrees that student nurses must demonstrate competence in areas such as professional values, communication and interpersonal skills, nursing practice and decision-making as well as leadership, management and team working before they become registered nurses (NMC 2010, p. 11). Their competence is judged by a sign-off mentor during the students' final clinical placement (NMC 2010). This places considerable responsibility on the sign-off mentor, whose assessment determines whether or not the student can work autonomously to deliver safe, compassionate and effective care as a qualified nurse.

The analytical eye – a one-dimensional vision of learning

We believe that a problem-solving approach alone over-develops the 'analytical eye' in the health practitioner and student. This is the first eye of the proposed three-eye model that we will examine in much more detail in Chapter 6. It is an incisive eye that sees a problem and defines a solution. Through this narrow focus, individuals take a detached and objective view that focuses on what is 'broken' or 'not working' and determines the best 'fix'.

We represent the analytical eye as a one-dimensional vision of learning and practice – a purely problem-solving approach that invites students and healthcare workers to define the solution and get to the answer. The care worker will, as part of a team, access the resources needed to gather the relevant background information and solve the presenting problem. The same process occurs in the educational context when looking at a case study or scenario. This type of self-directed PBL is a clear advance on the more traditional subject-based didactic teaching method because it involves an essential learning element. However, as we have seen, it is still a very limited approach. The problem, whether it is a trigger/scenario in teaching or one faced by the client in practice, is only seen from a detached, objective viewpoint. The focus is on the factual, technical, practical, measurable outcome. From an educational perspective, a critical appraisal and diagnosis is made of the situation, and the student judges what is needed to solve the problem. The goal is an intervention, whereby the student solves the problem by helping the client to adapt in some way.

However, what is commonly missed or devalued when using this approach is the role of the client in assessing and solving their own problem. The analytical problem-solving approach can become habitual and does not expand awareness to encompass the prospect of a more creative solution. By engaging in a self-directed, problem-solving approach whose goal is to find the problem and solve it, the students often takes sole responsibility for solving the problem. PBL is therefore, in essence, an approach to learning and problem solving that empowers the student and care worker to solve the client's problems for them. But does empowering the care worker to solve the problem, at the same time, disempower the client from fully engaging in solving their own problem? Could the care worker's good intentions actually be depriving the client of a vital source of learning?

Another limitation of a purely problem-solving approach is the narrow, partial and one-dimensional vision of the analytical eye. As we will explore more fully in Chapter 6, the analytical view is relatively superficial. The focus of our intervention, prior to taking action, influences the outcome that we find. Hawkins (2006, p. 237) reminds us that one's 'range of choice is ordinarily limited only by one's vision'. In line with this view, Hammond (1998, p. 6) notes that if 'we look only for problems, then that's what we will find'. This implies that using only the analytical lens, which always looks for problems, inevitably results in the finding of more problems to be solved. Professions may thus become compulsively preoccupied with the act of problem solving.

Also, as we have seen, students using PBL can overlook the importance of 'what is working well' and may therefore miss the chance to engage the client in resolving their own problems (Machon 2005, Roberts 2010). Cloke and Goldsmith (2006, p. 179) raise a pertinent question: 'are we able to resist the narcotic of problem solving?' Hammond and Royal (1998, p. 9) note that 'we are obsessed with learning from our mistakes' but what about learning from our success? Do we always seek, whether knowing or unknowingly, to control the process? To what degree are we capable of letting things happen in a creative, relational way? Furthermore, might our habitual solving of problems inhibit a deeper possible learning of the client that is essential to their growth and development? If we can resist the temptation to urgently solve the problem, might we then engage students and ultimately the client more fully in the process (Machon 2005)? As Cloke and Goldsmith (2003, p. 180) put it, 'in thinking that we know the one correct answer and in deciding to enlarge our egos, we do so at the cost of reduced skills in the person who has to live with the result'.

Note that we are by no means denying the value of technical expertise, the vital, practical role of the highly skilled healthcare worker or the importance of problem solving. However, we are saying that this limited and partial viewpoint can sometimes unintentionally devalue the importance of the subjective tutor–student or practitioner–client relationship. The rationalising approach fostered by PBL can overshadow the importance of seeing the client as a whole person, beyond the immediate problem that they are presenting. In practice, we often find that the presenting problem is not in fact the most important problem for the client or the carer. So how can we find the ideal balance between applying technical expert skills and engaging more deeply in order to assess and appreciate the client's needs in a truly person-centred way? How important is the quality of the relationship that we build with the client? And to what degree should we engage the client in the process of solving their own problem?

As previously stated, PBL tends to keep students in their 'heads' and unaware of matters of 'the heart' (Machon 2005, Machon & Roberts 2010). By 'the heart', we mean a more appreciative and relational approach that engages the client's subjective experiences and desires. The analytical eye offers a dispassionate view, whereby the client is only known objectively (from the outside, looking in). Who they are and what they may need, as determined by their experience (from the inside, looking out), remains a mystery. This can foster a negative attitude and a culture in which the client is seen as 'a problem needing to be solved' and their fuller human potential is not recognised. Edmonstone (2006) notes how this focus on what is not working may lower morale by creating a sense of a problem-filled environment, when what we should be seeking is a satisfied client who is actively engaged and centrally involved in their own care.

The importance of person-centred care seems clear. Nevertheless, in everyday practice, it is undeniably difficult for healthcare practitioners to pursue this concept – in the face of massive workloads, time constraints and the common use of checklists that only focus on problem identification. Constant pressure to achieve 'more with less' simply compounds the problem. This situation does indeed create tensions, and makes us ask: how can we realise the espoused values of the NHS constitution? Working in this deficit-based culture and driven by the fear of not having enough time, the care worker can easily lose sight of the person as a whole. But our three-eye model was developed with this context in mind, and seeks to address care workers' essential need to respond, rather than react, to these very significant challenges.

Conclusion

The key limitation of a problem-solving approach in practice and education is therefore its predominantly analytical and rationalising method of addressing difficult situations and challenges. The analytical eye may blindly overlook the need to relate and more fully engage with the client in order to further their ownership of the problem and learning. This raises the key question: is this lens alone adequate and appropriate for the learning, practice and culture of healthcare? The next chapter will focus on the second perspective the student and care worker can adopt in practice, that of the 'appreciative eye'.

Chapter 4

Applying appreciative inquiry in practice and education

Introduction

This chapter will explore how appreciative inquiry (AI) can be effectively applied in healthcare practice and education. The intention is to show how the qualities underpinning AI as a concept can enhance the more traditional problem-solving approach in practice and education in order to add value and innovation. We will present the outcome of research studies that show AI's positive influence on how students think and how they approach problems in both professional practice and education. The expanded vision of the 'appreciative eye' (in contrast to that of the 'analytical eye') is discussed in more detail as the second dimension of the 'three-eye' model that is more fully elucidated in Chapter 6.

Inspired by Martin Seligman's concept of positive psychology and a consideration of strengths and virtues (Peterson & Seligman 2004), clinicians have become more aware that we need to help people, not just by working with their problems, but also by helping them develop well-being. This more positive and appreciative approach is increasingly being integrated into various therapies (Synder & Ingram 2006).

Our work recognises the value of the essential appreciative lens in practice and is influenced by literature that has emerged from the work of David Cooperrider and Diane Whitney, who are both regarded as pioneers in the development of AI (Cooperrider & Whitney 2005). Their research suggests that by focusing and building on perceptions of success, the AI approach assists affirmative individual and team working. People feel valued and empowered because they are sharing ownership of the organisational development, in this case healthcare. They affirm what works well in their professional environment; articulate the necessary goals required to achieve further success (Boyd & Bright 2007); and decide on an action plan to fulfil these goals (Fitzgerald *et al.* 2001), particularly with clients.

To achieve this, it is proposed that the practitioner poses the unconditional positive question so that clients and carers focus on the most life-giving, life-sustaining aspects of their experience. There are four stages in the process of building on success, affirming ideals and goals, and planning ahead, collectively known as the 4-D model (Cooperrider & Whitney 2000):

- Discovery – the first stage focuses on identifying the most positive aspects of the current experience
- Dream – the second stage identifies where ideal future development is envisioned, based on this experience
- Design – the third stage outlines where participants consolidate plans, and ways in which the ideal can be attained
- Destiny – the fourth and final stage affirms that the plans are put into practice, implementing the key action steps.

(Ludema et al. 2006)

The AI 4-D model will now be discussed in the context of its potential application in healthcare.

Appreciative inquiry – applied in practice

AI is reported to motivate and empower stakeholders to change their life, situation or organisation (Lewis, Passmore & Cantore 2008). Hammond and Royal (1998) believe the strengths of AI naturally balance the limitations of the problem-solving approach, namely an excessive focus on the negative challenge of the problem. Instead, AI emphasises the existence of a positive core in professional intervention and care – in other words, it focuses on the positive and on what is working well.

According to the AI approach, the source of previous success and strengths is a developmental organising principle – and the source of future growth. From this perspective, development and learning are a natural consequence of identifying success and what is, and has been, working well for the client. According to this approach, any problem should initially be studied within the larger context of what is working well. This significantly expands the understanding of the impact of the problem and therefore informs its resolution. AI is a way of working to bring about positive change that concentrates on 'the best in people, their organisations, and the world around them' (Cooperrider & Whitney 2005, p. 8).

Whereas a problem-solving approach places emphasis objectively on finding the problem, AI focuses subjectively on the value and importance of relationship to learning and growth. As discussed previously, problem solving employs the partial vision and characteristics of the 'analytical eye', whereas AI requires the opening of what we describe as the 'appreciative eye'. If care workers can learn to combine both viewpoints, their vision, practice, care and learning can be markedly developed. We need to cultivate a more integrated and creative vision – what we describe in our model as 'a creative eye' – that naturally accommodates both the analytical and appreciative aspects. This invites care workers, students and tutors alike to use both viewpoints to realise a multi-dimensional integrative vision.

Even though problem solving and AI can be seen as two opposing and starkly contrasting learning approaches, one in fact complements the other, and this view is explored in more detail in Chapter 6. They can actually be seen less as two opposing approaches to learning and more as 'two sides of the same coin' of learning (Machon & Roberts 2010). In embracing this concept, tutors, students and healthcare workers can allow a more creative and relational approach to practice, learning and teaching. Machon (2010, p. 139) refers to this as 'paradox in practice' and suggests that paradox is a 'portal to a deeper appreciation of reality and a knowledge that guides us close to remembering our original self'. The value of such a paradox is that it reminds us of the potential of a more unlimited vision and fosters our capacity to include both a relational and rational approach in practice. This concept is illustrated and discussed in more detail in Chapters 5 and 7, where we consider creativity and mindfulness in practice.

We propose that initially building on perceptions of success, rather than focusing on failure, can help us attain improvements in professional healthcare practice more easily. This approach necessarily involves an appreciative engagement of the client. Based on these principles, AI as a model of intervention and research encourages organisational development through effective group discussion and collaborative and respectful teamwork. In a study looking at the application of AI in practice, Clarke and Thornton (2014, p. 475) reported an increase in confidence and improved experiences, with 'AI providing a guiding structure and a framework that enhanced and sustained positive change'.

In large national and international corporate organisations, including the NHS in the UK, AI has been seen as a major breakthrough in organisational development, training and problem-solving. In this context, AI is based on the assertion that problems are often partly the result of our own perspectives and perceptions. For example, if we look at a certain priority as a problem, we tend to constrain our ability to address that priority effectively.

AI is actually a philosophy, from which a variety of models, tools and techniques can be derived. For example, one AI-based approach to strategic planning includes the following key steps:

- Identifying our best times during the best situations in the past
- Thinking about what worked best then
- Envisioning what we want in the future
- Building on what worked best in the past to work towards our vision for the future.

This approach has arguably revolutionised many practices, including strategic planning, leadership and organisational development.

In a study by Roberts (2010), professionals with advanced specialist knowledge in mental health, for example, shifted their focus from problem solving to AI in a very tangible way. Traditionally, mental health work has been more rooted in a social model of care than a medical model. Many believe that mental health has already made its own shift, from the study of pathology (analytical) to the study of the conditions and processes that contribute to optimum function (appreciative). In this sense, a clear link can be made between the underlying principles of AI and those of positive psychology. It is therefore appropriate to endorse positive psychology in this context. Applying psychology in practice, learning and teaching is not only about the study of pathology, weakness and damage but also the study of strengths and virtues, another potential endorsement of the principles of AI.

We have argued already, in Chapter 3, that an over-emphasis on the habitual, problem-solving analytical eye can lead to the negative impact of unconscious care. By this we mean that standards may drop, we may become uncaring, we may rush things, and potentially forget the human element – essentially becoming 'heart-less'. As we have seen, the analytical lens is incisive and focuses purely on the problem and impulsively defining the solution. By focusing on problem solving alone, healthcare workers and students may take a detached and objective viewpoint that looks for what is 'broken'. Yet the limitations inherent in problem solving actually create an opportunity for the natural evolution of a complementary practice and learning approach – that of AI (Machon & Roberts 2010).

This highlights the need to apply AI more proactively and consciously in practice and education in order to meet the recommendations of the Francis Report (2013). AI can play a key role in enhancing and promoting quality in professional healthcare practice. This idea is supported by Rubin *et al.* (2011, p. 236), whose research into AI reminds the care worker that 'AI changes focus from the practitioner to the client'. The Rubin study also observed that 'clients benefited from the focus on their own wishes rather than what the therapist believed would be advantageous' (p. 236). Implementing AI in practice may therefore enhance an affirmative person-centred practice and more collaborative working. Clinicians and practice educators who participated in the Rubin study stressed the importance of maximising their own positive attitudes as a basis for creating more powerful social experiences to help students discover the best about themselves, and how they saw clients, colleagues and team working. This principle is fundamental in ensuring that healthcare students move towards an appreciative perspective on themselves and their situation. Equally, if educators and students start using more appreciative language when speaking about clients, clinical situations and team working it will help them build a more balanced view of themselves.

Increasingly, AI is being incorporated into undergraduate healthcare university courses to help ensure that curricula delivery is fit for purpose. New healthcare graduates entering professional practice must be equipped to meet the requirements of clients, colleagues and the wider organisation in a very demanding and rapidly changing environment. Integrating AI with more traditional pedagogies (such as PBL) will significantly contribute to students' success in meeting such challenges.

Appreciative inquiry – applied in education

When an academic tutor and practice educator builds on the traditional PBL approach by proactively guiding students to start using AI, the students usually show a more positive attitude and approach. We are reminded once again that our range of choice is ordinarily limited only by our vision. With PBL, there is a danger that the students' potential preoccupation with problem solving and getting to the answer may prevent them from taking a more expansive view of the scenario and/or client. Historically, there has been an apparent obsession with learning from mistakes but, by resisting the temptation to solve the problem with urgency, educators can attempt to engage the student (and in turn the client) more fully in the process.

Another potential danger of PBL is that in thinking we know the one correct answer we do so at the cost of reduced skills in the person who has to live with the result. This is not to deny the very practical role of the healthcare practitioner or student to problem-solve. However, the PBL approach, whereby solutions to a problem are based on past experiences of self and others, can lead to us only seeing the presented problem and not the client as a person.

In a qualitative study of academic tutors' perceptions of PBL, almost all the participants expressed concern that there can be too much emphasis on diagnosis-led outcomes within PBL (Roberts 2013). This in turn tends to drive healthcare students towards predetermined solutions, rather than looking for a more creative and person-centred approach as central to the problem-solving process. The focus on problem solving is seen by some tutors as a barrier that prevents the students from focusing creatively on more person-centred care.

There is also some criticism of the medical model that apparently sees human systems as machines and only views clients in a partial way. At times, it seems that healthcare workers can only enable individuals to adapt to their problematic situation. But when a given problem cannot be solved, the practitioner can use their knowledge and skill not only to help the client adapt to the problem but also to live a full, meaningful and purposeful life.

Case study (Part 2)

In the Roberts (2013) study, an image scenario was given to three first-year PBL groups in occupational therapy (as described in Chapter 2). Students were asked to reflect on a photograph showing a dishevelled young man, with long hair, cradling an old dog in the doorway of a high-street shop on a rainy day. He was holding an empty cup of coffee. He spoke to no one, just looked down.

Meanwhile, three other groups of students followed a newly developed problem-solving/appreciative inquiry cycle. These students were asked to reflect on the same photographic image and identify their learning needs. No associated verbal or written prompts were given, so these students also had to make many assumptions.

This experiment was also carried out with similar groups four years in succession, and the results were consistent across all groups.

As stated the first set of assumptions that informed the learning needs identified by the groups were:
- The individual was homeless.
- He had associated mental health problems.
- He had associated drug and alcohol problems.
- His behaviour was manipulative because he was using the dog to get money to feed his habit.
- He had poor hygiene and personal care.
- He was a societal nuisance.
- He was occupationally deprived.
- This was an example of abuse of the welfare state.

However, these three groups also applied AI and identified the following additional and more affirming questions and learning needs:
- If homeless, is he there by choice or by circumstances?
- What is his human potential?
- What has he achieved?
- As a carer for the dog, is he occupationally engaged?
- If perceived to be dishevelled, by whose standards?
- Where is the evidence that he has poor personal hygiene?
- Is he a problem to himself or others?
- Where does his personal choice lie?

These combined PBL/AI groups also took a very anti-stereotypical view of this image, stating that there was:
- No evidence of mental health problems
- No evidence of drug or alcohol abuse
- No evidence that the welfare system was being abused
- No evidence of poor hygiene.

Having evaluated the learning needs and outcomes resulting from this new approach, these students also identified some negative attitudes and assumptions from the PBL focus. However, it is very noticeable that they also considered more affirmative and less biased and stereotypical learning needs. They did not make assumptions based on seeing the image as a problem to be solved. Instead, these students saw human potential. They asked different questions and made fewer negative assumptions. Overall, their assessment of this image was predominantly positive, more person-centred, less judgemental and more appreciative. Clearly, these students had expanded their thinking by opening an appreciative eye.

Concern has sometimes been expressed at the way in which some students perceive their future role in healthcare (McKenna & Supyk 2006). Inherent in PBL are negative and judgemental assumptions about life, people, and the process of change itself, as it affects clients and their families. Yet a move away from a focus on problem solving sometimes appears to disturb or unsettle student groups. Other students may be happy to see their role as facilitating a more person-centred, collaborative and appreciative approach.

In any context (whether it be in a society, an organisation, a multi-disciplinary team, a group, in a community or with an individual), something is likely to be working well. This all-inclusive view reflects a person-centred approach and the values that should underpin practice and care, a perception that is promising for those who facilitate the education of the future healthcare workforce. Should PBL facilitators therefore search for ways to shift the prevailing strategy away from fixing problems (which may or may not make a situation better) and towards discovering what individuals or organisations want their lives to be? Instead of focusing on what is not working in their triggers, groups or clinical practice, students could then begin to explore what gave people happiness and fulfilment when they were at their very best. Should tutors and students start daring to ask questions about hope and aspiration, and begin to see people not as problems to be solved but as miracles and mysteries to be appreciated?

The relationship between AI and PBL

Note that the apparent limitations of the traditional model of PBL are not concerned with its problem-solving process but more its context and partial vision. Through effective facilitation, tutors can help students to suspend these habits. Approaching PBL with an open mind and heart offers students an opportunity to see learning triggers/scenarios with fresh, inquiring, reflective and more appreciative eyes. It also encourages the development of empathy and helps students to navigate difficulties in a more positive frame of mind – not from a place of anxiety to solve, but from a place of excitement and potential creativity.

Healthcare workers and educators should challenge the traditional focus on pure problem solving because focusing on the problem alone has the effect of devaluing the individual client and limiting creative therapeutic intervention. Shifting to AI will change professional practice and attitudes towards care. It will also dilute the tendency to view the human condition as a machine, which when broken has to be fixed. This attitude may well show a characteristic human desire to solve, but it also prevents us from seeing the full human condition. Looking at a situation with an appreciative eye may provide an added element to PBL, one in which healthcare workers and students alike may focus more on the positive aspects of a particular situation. This approach, when applied in practice and learning, can help individuals to consider their previous experience and re-use positive outcomes. Practice educators, in particular, could facilitate a positive approach to ensure that students engage themselves in the educational process and use such transferable skills in practice.

The appreciative eye – a two-dimensional vision of learning

We are now clear that our compulsive problem solving is a consequence of an active 'analytical eye', whereas AI necessitates the opening of what we describe as the 'appreciative eye'. This is the second of the three eyes in the model that we examine in more detail in Chapter 6. If the healthcare student or worker can employ the appreciative lens in a conscious way, the quality of care, vision, practice and learning can be significantly expanded. Even though problem solving and AI can be seen as two starkly contrasting approaches to practice and education, one in fact complements the other and both are necessary to the best-quality caring. In embracing this, care workers and students can take a more creative and relational approach to learning, teaching and professional practice. This blended approach reminds us all of the importance of a more unlimited vision, and fosters our capacity to work both rationally and relationally in a more compassionate and caring way. Thus, we can integrate an incisive and decisive practical approach with a more appreciative and relational practice.

This opening of the appreciative eye in the care worker reflects what we might term 'an opening of the heart', giving a more empathic and potentially compassionate focus. In this way, care workers and healthcare students shift from just seeing a problem to viewing the individual as they see themselves. The role of the practitioner as a facilitator of care then becomes central to the client's and/or student's learning experience.

The challenges of appreciative inquiry

Building positive connections and engagement requires us to move from focusing on problems to using more appreciative language. In doing this, students and practitioners will learn to reframe their problem-solving perspectives and negative self-talk to be more affirmative. However, one of the challenges of AI is the language and terminology used in the original '4D' model. Many people find words like 'discovery', 'dreams', 'design' and 'destiny' (Cooperrider & Srivastva 1987) rather vague and open to a variety of interpretations. Making sense of AI language can therefore become a challenge in itself and this issue may need to be addressed by those who choose to build on its potential in practice and learning.

AI is an expansive, relational and empathic learning approach so the use of such expansive and ungrounded terms is understandable. However, pertinent language is important in order to gain acceptance of this approach and time must therefore be invested in thinking about alternative, more specific terms to use in practice and learning environments. Initial thoughts, for example, have leant towards substitutes for some of these terms. For instance, 'discovery' can be replaced by 'inquiry', 'dream' by 'imagine', 'design' by 'innovate' and 'destiny' by 'implement'.

Some of this discussion may sound abstract and academic – and perhaps somewhat distant from those on the frontline of everyday practice. It should be remembered that much of our community care is given by unsupervised care workers employed independently, including those working with the chronically ill, the disabled and those in palliative care. These care workers are also largely responsible for the feeding, washing and toileting of hospitalised patients. It is essential to reach them and influence their thinking around appreciative and compassionate care. The three-eye model is as relevant to them as it is to any other practitioner, since compassion and care go together as priorities in any care strategy, irrespective of the individual care worker's position in the organisational hierarchy.

Conclusion

In our view, it is by no means chance that AI is emerging as a contrasting valuable and insightful approach to healthcare practice and learning. The limitations of PBL have in fact informed the emergent strengths of learning through AI. As we have seen, these two approaches are naturally complementary. AI invites the teacher or practitioner to become more aware of, and to engage with and discover, a 'positive core'. This is a source of the student's and client's potential learning, growth, motivation and aspiration, and therefore indicates the desired direction of their future success and potential fulfilment.

The invitation through AI is to relate to the client in order to appreciate their success, passions and future aspirations. This deeper, more relational and subjective awareness offers a fertile context in which to consider the apparent 'problem' that they face and how it might best be resolved.

Key to the evolution of learning and practice is how we can support the use of these new approaches in healthcare practice and education. Coaching and supervisory support may be needed in order to maximise learning and growth, and the value of these support systems is discussed in Chapters 7 and 8 respectively. Jung (1938, p. 15) noted that 'the greatest and most important problems in life are all in a certain sense insoluble. They must be so because they express the necessary polarity inherent in every self-regulating system. They can never be solved… only outgrown'. This insight points towards a deeper paradox within our concept of the problem. If we could view problems as a source of personal learning, could they in fact foster our growth? It seems that the urgency to solve problems may deprive us of the chance to learn and grow through exploring those very problems.

In the next chapter, we explore the concept of creativity applied in healthcare, as a natural progression and evolution of our thinking. We challenge the reader to promote creative thinking and practice as a way of enhancing affirmative innovation in all aspects of professional work and specifically in the way we care.

Chapter 5

Creativity and care

Introduction

Chapters 3 and 4 have presented two perspectives of the 'three-eye' model – those of the analytical and appreciative eye. In this chapter we will introduce the third perspective, that of the 'creative eye', and then progress to view the relationship between all three eyes in more detail in Chapter 6.

Defining creativity and its application in healthcare is both complex and difficult. There is often some confusion about the use of the word 'creativity' because it is an abstract concept (Worth 2000). It is also a relative and context-dependent concept (Hart 2000). Worth (2000) further suggests that creativity is a fundamental human attribute that helps us adapt and respond to a fast-changing and sometimes dangerous world.

Pause and reflect

- What is your understanding of creativity in practice?
- Do you consider yourself to be a creative person? Reflect on times in which you
- have recognised your own creative potential, or have been complimented by others on coming up with a new or innovative idea.
- Do you recognise creativity in others? If so, do you acknowledge the person's creativity?

Care workers need to consciously focus not only on promoting their specialist knowledge in their chosen clinical or professional field, but also on utilising creative and lateral thinking in all aspects of their caring role. A conscientious and mindful practitioner is likely to be creative in many different ways. For example, they:

- Approach caring differently, with an open mind
- See beyond the immediate situation by redefining the presenting problem
- Produce something that is new

- Maximise opportunities to engage in novel and useful approaches to open-ended tasks
- Aspire to achieve something that is affirmative and opportunistic
- Become an effective team player, leader and manager of themselves and others.

The creative care worker can enhance their awareness, personal qualities and professional abilities by:

- Showing genuine and mindful interest in others
- Attending to needs in an open and engaging way
- Addressing problem-solving with both analytical and appreciative lenses
- Responding creatively and adaptively to each scenario
- Having high self-esteem and confidence
- Having innovative and affirmative problem-solving skills
- Being intrinsically rather than extrinsically motivated
- Understanding the true nature of professionalism
- Showing a natural and unconditional approach to vulnerability.

Riley and Matheson (2010) reflect on the complex challenges of enhancing such qualities in individuals of different ages, genders, interests, abilities and intellects. Wider access to courses means that students often come from very diverse cultural, social and educational backgrounds. Some training programmes, such as those for the allied health professions, nursing or social work, where professional or accreditation bodies demand particular curricula content, may emphasise diagnosis-led problem-solving outcomes. This may push students towards predetermined solutions, rather than encouraging them to adopt a more creative and person-centred approach (Riley & Matheson 2010). Some graduates, on entering their first professional post, may not therefore be trained in a truly person-centred way.

A creative person responds positively, adaptively and, according to Riley and Matheson (2010), sees beyond the immediate situation and is able to redefine complex problems. These attributes are considered important in a rapidly changing healthcare environment and culture. Mindful engagement with AI, as an approach to problem solving in a person-centred manner, offers practitioners the opportunity to develop such qualities, which characterise the motivated carer. With the knowledge and skill to question and understand the complexity of everyday situations, professional carers and students alike can face the challenges they encounter in a more affirmative, creative and person-centred way.

Characteristics of creativity in practice

Approaching care in a creative and mindful way is likely to lead to a better understanding of values and norms that in turn encourage critical thinking and questioning, open exploration, reformulation, originality and innovation. This process can be facilitated by a conscious awareness of how professional practice is approached and the extent to which we can influence our professional and caring intervention through creative thinking. An effective manager or leader may therefore need to consider devoting time to supervise or even coach colleagues to seek out alternative perspectives, reformulate problems and further develop their imagination and intuitive ability. Understanding the process of creativity in the context of problem solving may well be a way of facilitating achievement in a specific caring or clinical task.

Creativity and the human condition

What model best represents our understanding of ourselves? Each and every one of us is a being that is forever in the process of becoming more developed (Whiteford & Wilcock 2002). Machon (2008, p. 37) recognises this when he invites us to 'participate in the creative mystery of becoming'. As human beings, we have a number of key motivations, including the drive to creatively problem-solve and the aspiration to become something more than we are.

AI includes a consideration of what is working well and also a problem-solving element, combining both positive and negative viewpoints. The key question is: how can we combine both a problem-solving and a more appreciative approach, to include the aspirations and wishes of the client, affirming their present being, whilst also recognising their vital aspiration to take practical steps forward in order to become more complete? Such an approach would accommodate the client's multiple potential drives, their present being and their desire to develop. Consider how the care worker can marry the present being and reality of the client with their future aspirations to implement their desired change.

To bring the client's present reality into focus, we might ask:

- What is working well?
- What has worked well previously?
- What does success look like?
- Is there a problem?
- What is the problem?
- How might we best attempt to solve it?

To identify their future aspirations, we could ask:
- What brings you joy and makes your 'heart sing'?
- How might this help you through this period?
- What do you aspire to?
- What would you ideally like to happen?
- Who do you ideally want to be and become?

Such an approach to learning and practice, which embraces both the individual's being and becoming, can be described as 'paradoxical inquiry' (Machon & Roberts 2010). Gathering this spectrum of information from the client and/or carer provides a much more complete, authentic and person-centred picture, including their desire for change and what will motivate that change. It respects the innate paradoxical nature of the client and considers both their current state and future aspirations. Taking such an appreciative and creative stance can potentially be about searching for the best in people, in the NHS as a system, and in the political and economic world around them. In its broadest focus, it involves systematic discovery of what gives energy to a system when it is most alive, most effective, and most capable in environmental, economic, ecological and human terms.

An appreciative approach essentially involves asking questions that strengthen a system's capacity to apprehend, anticipate and heighten positive potential. It expands awareness through inquiry and application of appreciative questioning. The actual steps of this process are considered in much more detail in Chapter 8, where we explore the nature of the coaching conversation. Taking forward such an appreciative approach highlights the fact that our ability to care is heavily influenced by our capacity for positive regard, imagination and innovation, rather than negation, criticism and diagnosis. By utilising AI as a creative approach, care workers can aspire to achieve the following personal and professional qualities and goals:

- Recognising their own successes and achievements
- Acknowledging their past and present capacities
- Discovering their personal assets
- Realising their unexplored potential
- Being innovative
- Recognising their signature strengths
- Intuitive realisations and Eureka moments
- Realising opportunities
- Living according to their values

- Discovering empowering beliefs
- Being able to adopt a strategic context
- Expressing wisdom
- Gaining spiritual insights
- Realising their vision of an ideal future
- Recognising their innate resourcefulness.

Pause and reflect

- In your daily personal and professional life, how often do you acknowledge the above qualities and aspirations in yourself and others?
- In your caring role, how often do you ask your clients these questions?

Creativity and paradox

It is important to consider our creativity in the context of both personal and organisational flourishing and how we may utilise our creative selves to stay ahead of the game – in the public, private and voluntary sectors. Creativity can be a source of competitive strength within organisations such as the NHS and Local Authorities who have faced stressful and chaotic conditions for some time, under various governments.

However, it is also important to remember that there is no magic formula for creativity. It is only possible to identify the factors that make creative behaviours and attitudes within a caring role more likely. These factors may include:

- Establishing a culture, leadership style and value system that encourage professionals to think and act beyond their current wisdom
- Concentrating more on informal structures and lines of communications than their formal equivalents
- Ensuring that the built environment is comfortable, fit for purpose and stimulating
- Devising systems of reward, recognition and personal growth that fit with the strategy of continuing professional development and advancement.

Pause and reflect

- Consider your own working or study environment. How conducive is it to creative thinking?
- What can you and your team do to make it better?
- If you were in charge, how would it be different?

If the rational mind can be taught to be patient and to accept the paradoxes we face (rather than compulsively trying to solve them), both clients and practitioners may find that they are able to reflect upon problems and dilemmas more creatively. Without this problem-solving pressure, practitioners may be free to relate more fully to each other and their clients in practice, both recognising who the person is now and who they long to become. In our ability to reflect and question, we recall the larger context and accommodate our vital aspirations. Problems then become less of an obstacle to be solved and more explicitly a guide to our desire for growth and learning.

Paradoxically, we can learn through our problems. A problem is also an opportunity and a prospect – that is, if we can resist the temptation to solve it straight away. As practitioners, we may need to realise that questions are just as important as answers. It is through questions that we enable our clients' aspirations to be consciously expressed. A quick solution closes a door on the chance to reflect upon the vital questions lying beneath the superficial problem. By opting for a 'quick fix', we may in fact exacerbate the real problem rather than alleviating it. Paradox teaches us that there is value in being able to both expand and contract our awareness, and having the capacity to both question and answer.

Indeed, a vision of caring through either the analytical and or appreciative eye will in itself be limited. We propose that there is greater value in integrating both aspects to accommodate a much more responsive and unlimited vision – that of the creative eye. What additional value might we find if we could combine the best of the PBL and AI approaches, rather than applying them as distinct and separate entities? In this way, we could make problem solving less of a compulsion and more of a choice, empowering the client to learn and grow by actively engaging with, and helping to resolve, their own problems.

Creatively managing multi-disciplinary teams and processes

Attending to the more mystifying dimensions of team working in healthcare environments can be a much more challenging task than managing the more familiar and tangible aspects. Unexpressed anxieties or fears can be destructive in any work relationship and may have dire effects on how we consciously (or not) care for clients, ourselves and our colleagues. It may sometimes seem easier to keep quiet, turn a blind eye and avoid appearing disloyal or looking foolish or unprofessional.

'Whistleblowing' has been a 'taboo' discussion point within teams for a long time. Roberts (2010) outlined the impact of the Kennedy Report in 2001 as well as the drive for clinical governance and the need to report poor practice. Yet the very fact that information is often withheld creates a separation between the people concerned. As care professionals, managers and leaders, we must create a safe, non-judgemental and trusting environment in which individuals feel able to express and hear anxieties. It is often the 'hands on', frontline practitioners who feel silenced by management, whilst facing the pressure to meet targets and work at the 'coal face'.

How can we promote the development of a culture that supports the courageous individual in stepping forward and voicing their concerns, despite being faced with issues of silencing and lack of trust? Mindful of the highlighted importance of compassion, care and courage in the healthcare strategic agenda, can we now expect to see more leaders, managers and care workers having the courage to act and speak out when essential values are ignored?

Pause and reflect

- If you have suspicions or fears of mis-care, neglect and or abuse, what would you do about reporting or dealing with it?
- What would help you to take this important step?

In a culture of increasing litigation and accountability, managing a complex organisation and multi-disciplinary teams is not easy. It usually involves an on-going process, with its own frustrations, lessons and breakthroughs. Rather than team building workshops, what is also often required is a sustained awareness of the human concerns present in any group of people, and the ability to handle the team process. Within these more subtle and personal team dynamics, there may be a need to bring elements of the creative process to bear. Care workers do not usually come together as a team immediately; they generally need an initial period of preparation and induction. There may be periods of anxiety and frustration as team members begin to understand their roles and find their place, agree professional boundaries and address unresolved issues in a complex environment. Evans and Russell (1989) recognise that there needs to be a receptive working environment in order to facilitate insights and breakthroughs.

In such a rapidly changing organisation as the NHS there is much that can be done to facilitate the inner aspects – not only of the team process but also the interface between carer and client. This may mean that teams need to consider:

- Setting aside time for individuals to talk about how they are, what they are feeling, and, when appropriate, their hopes and fears, and any issues that may be challenging them.
- Allowing time for team members to settle and feel at ease, and be heard and accepted as part of the team. This may even be more important when introducing undergraduate students to their practice experience.

- Creating a climate in which the team can work more smoothly and tackle more effectively any managerial issues that arise.
- Encouraging others to share their anxieties, concerns and issues, in the knowledge that giving such permission allows plans and agendas to be put on the table in an open and trustworthy way.
- Above all, approaching other people's needs, feelings and concerns with the sensitivity, care and compassion with which you would like your own to be handled.

All organisations need effective self-management and respectful teamwork – and none more so than those operating within the care sector. This is relevant to all levels of management, from the chief executive to the therapist, to the support worker, to the ward nurse. Evans and Russell (1989) believe that most organisations place team-building high on their agendas. Various experiments have been tried, and important insights have been gained in understanding how individuals and teams work. Many different theories and models have been developed, and there are now several different methods of exploring individual roles and team profiles. Yet, despite this continuing investment of time and energy, getting a multi-disciplinary team to gel and work effectively is still a mysterious process. And if such a team fails to work as it should, the potential impact on client care in a health service can be disastrous.

Much of the work on team-building has focused on social issues, but there are deeper personal issues that may also need to be addressed. In healthcare these personal issues are seldom voiced, often difficult to observe, and frequently hidden by fear and anxiety. Even when they are revealed, both clients and professionals have still often – as recent history has shown – felt unheard and ignored.

Society tends to regard these elusive and mysterious human traits as weaknesses and personal foibles. We generally expect colleagues to act without hidden agendas or personal biases – that is, we hope they will be perfectly rational and supportive team members. Unfortunately, this ideal may not be prevalent in practice. This is not to imply that some textbook models are ineffective, only that they are partial. Evans and Russell (1989) believe that it is equally important to learn to manage the more unpredictable human processes that are found in every team and in every organisation, and none more so than the care sector. Managing such complex individuals and teams requires clear structures for supervision, mentoring and coaching. Supervision and coaching in healthcare are discussed further in Chapter 8.

As well as technical skill, supervision needs to employ a high degree of relational and rational intelligence. The role of the tutor in cultivating learning is shifting from one of instructor and technical expert to one of facilitator and coach. Those of us who supervise others need to accommodate and appreciate this shifting role and the importance of our ability to coach and facilitate in order to maximise our own and our client's learning. How much more fulfilled might our clients and practitioners be if we could truly implement this approach to practice and learning in healthcare? This type of supervision would value our clients' fulfilment and learning as highly as the more measurable outcomes of our expert technical practice. Machon and Roberts (2010) believe that this evolving vision might inspire a culture that supports both our continued learning and best practice.

When attempting to devise approaches that will increase the potential for creativity to ensure positive change, it is vital to take into account the richness and potential of differing organisational cultures, varying leadership styles, structures, systems, values, beliefs, resources and knowledge/skill base, in addition to outlining the importance of facilitation as a skill that enables creative change to occur.

Facilitation and creative change

Facilitation is viewed by Barrows (2002) as a dynamic goal-orientated process, in which participants work together in an atmosphere of mutual respect, and learn through critical reflection. Facilitation is thus seen as person-centred and collaborative: a process of synthesis involving shared learning and the development of critical thinking. However, the actual role of the facilitator remains elusive and only vaguely specified (Haith-Cooper 2000). This may well be partly because of the individual and subjective way in which each professional perceives facilitation. Rogers (1983, p. 189) maintained that a facilitator creates 'an atmosphere of realness, of caring and of understanding listening', and that this enhances the learning and practice environments. Facilitators may therefore need to find a balance – striving for a style and skill base that promotes client satisfaction and meets individual and group needs, while also maintaining the boundaries and outcomes created by the organisation in which they work.

Facilitating positive and creative change invites the care worker to enter a collaborative learning relationship with their client. In this context, the care worker's role requires:

- The ability to create a climate for learning
- The flexibility to cope with changing agendas
- The capability to respond to individual needs
- The capacity to engage clients and colleagues in reflective dialogue and critical thinking.

By adopting a reflective approach in practice, healthcare facilitators get an opportunity to explore their own actions and develop a level of self-awareness and responsiveness to others that is key to proactive change. Similarly, peer review systems and support from other colleagues are ways of enhancing our understanding of how to facilitate creatively. Placing the client at the very heart of decisions may offer an opportunity for direct feedback and consequently give the client an opportunity to be heard. This may not only offer a more equitable partnership but also enhance the client's sense of self-worth when their voice is valued. In Chapter 8 we will examine how these facilitation skills can be utilised in the work of a coach in a healthcare setting.

The challenges of compassionate care are often dealt with in one of two ways – either automatic and prescriptively or specifically based on the client's present need by creating opportunities, based on the client's personal experience, to realise the desired change. A creative and conscientious care worker endeavours to guide the client into their own experience, to expand their awareness and encourage them to participate in the caring process. Such learning experiences can give meaning to the vocation of caring. It is more respectful and creative for the practitioner to involve the client as a whole person in interaction and inquiry by getting them to participate in their own development, learning and resolution of desired goals.

We ask, in the care worker's urgent need to solve problems, do we over-simplify and miss the vital chance to contemplate and learn more deeply from the dilemma presented? Might the appreciation of these deeper dilemmas guide team members towards a more creative, elegant and balanced solution? The analytical eye is always intent on critically judging what is 'right' or 'wrong' and so simplifying the potential of problem solving as a creative process. Paradox, with its innate contradiction, suggests that there may always be more than one possibility and there could be wisdom in considering more than just the 'either/or'.

Paradox is not to be reductively resolved. It should be seen more in terms of the potential it offers for learning to be fully embraced. If care workers can learn to expand their vision to see, value and accept the paradoxical nature of the creative lens, might they also learn how to extend their thinking beyond the critical and rational? Paradox, if owned, may provide a secret alchemy that can transform the urgency to solve into a deeper, more imaginative and creative curiosity (Machon 2005). An appreciation of creative paradox uniquely offers a dynamic flexibility of response, with an ability to balance alongside it the capacity to both relate and/or solve, as required. This awareness offers the care worker the possibility of a much more flexible, innovative and creative response.

When we integrate these learning approaches, there is a major shift in the quality of our practice and learning. The chance to expand awareness allows the practitioner to verify whether this is the key problem faced by the client, how the client might engage and learn through the solving of the problem, and how the client's aspirations might reframe and inform the problem. This places an initial emphasis on the AI approach and primarily engaging the 'appreciative eye' in order to relate to the client more deeply. Problem solving is still important but becomes less central. The approach becomes less problem-focused and more solution-focused, and the care worker's technical skills are married with the personal understanding and expertise of the client. In this context, the presenting problem finds its true value and meaning. From this relational perspective, the practitioner can further engage with the client to explore how they themselves may wish to resolve the problem. Having established this breadth and scope of information, relative to the presenting problem, the healthcare worker can then engage the 'analytical eye' more consciously to plan the most practical next steps.

Two key realisations emerge through an appreciation of our deeper paradoxical nature. Firstly, our awareness of the problem is expanded through different ways of seeing, sensing and thinking, thus extending the client and practitioner's capacity for learning. Secondly, there is the discovery of a more creative and compassionate solution. Throughout, this approach ensures that the client (rather than the care worker) is centrally empowered in the process of finding solutions to their care, whilst continuing to learn and develop.

Finally, we have realised that it is vital to be open to such paradox in a way that provides an attentive and listening ear. Giving such attention offers a rare opportunity for discussion of limitations as well as strengths. We believe such openness is a key that can unlock learning potential.

Conclusion

In all aspects of healthcare, the 'analytical eye' is always focused on finding the answer. When care workers employ the analytical eye, they take on the role of an instructor. The inclusion of the 'appreciative eye' shifts the role of the practitioner from one of a reactive problem-solver to more of a questioning and listening facilitator. Rather than seeking the answer, the opening of the 'appreciative eye' gives the practitioner the chance to explore the value of the question. In addition, the 'appreciative eye' is a sensing as well as a seeing eye; it is keen to listen as well as observe and so it is able to relate with true empathy. The vision of the 'appreciative eye' therefore extends awareness beyond the self to embrace a deeper appreciation of the other.

As a learning approach, this may encourage students to maximise the value of learning through the student–tutor relationship. This integrative approach to learning develops our capacity to listen, and enhances our ability to relate to each other as team members, and to our clients, as well as making us aware of the need (at the appropriate time) to focus, solve and decide. A deeper learning can be gained by consciously working with both the 'analytical and appreciative eyes', whilst fully engaging the client in their own care.

As we have discussed, this further step happens through the opening of the 'creative eye'. The 'creative eye' looks beyond the limitations of the 'either/or' to engage both 'the either and the or' and potentially still something more. Both the analytical and appreciative aspects of our awareness are employed, and in addition we have a dynamic flexibility to listen, question, relate and resolve. Once more, this defines the work of the care worker and coach as examined in detail in Chapter 8.

To understand this innovative approach, and further explore its application in practice and learning, Chapter 6 will look at what we call the 'three-eye model'. This model offers a more person-centred approach to healthcare practice and learning and guides us in how to become more responsive carers. In the next chapter, we more fully introduce the application of the 'three eye model' to healthcare education and practice. We will examine the key characteristics of the analytical, appreciative and creative lenses respectively, and how the vision of each lens influences the care worker's capability and approach.

Chapter 6

Applying the three-eye model to healthcare

Introduction

The aim of this chapter is to introduce in detail the 'three-eye model' and its full potential in practice and education. It will also examine the key characteristics of the analytical, appreciative and creative eyes respectively and how our approach to practice changes markedly, depending on the position and perspective we take.

The 'three-eye model' may at first appear an unfamiliar concept. Very simply, this model acknowledges that the vision of the carer is not fixed, though we may think it so. We can consciously adopt different viewpoints that expand our awareness and vision of caring and, in doing so, permit ourselves to develop important qualities and skills. The 'three eyes' can be seen as three different lenses that collectively comprise our full vision as a carer. This terminology allows us to highlight important distinctions as we move from one lens to another. We invite the reader to approach these concepts with an open mind despite their unfamiliarity in order to gain the full benefit and learning. Primarily, we explore the application of the 'three-eye model' to the individual carer but it can equally well be applied to the work of a multi-disciplinary healthcare team. It allows a deeper awareness of, and respect for, the shared skills and resources of the team. It also opens the way to a collaborative and compassionate approach to patient care that can be maintained and sustained through the operation of the team.

As previously stated, we cannot ignore the impact of the Francis Report (2013), which revealed an insidious negative culture involving a tolerance of poor standards, a disengagement from key responsibilities, and a lack of basic kindness and care. Questions continue to be asked as to how such a profound lack of care, neglect and even client abuse could happen in an establishment whose primary responsibility is to offer safe, high-quality care. Here, we respond to these questions by illustrating how the 'three-eye model' can offer us new insight into how any one of us can become uncaring in practice. This awareness can guide us in discovering how to deliver and sustain person-centred care. In today's healthcare system, many interactions with patients will clearly be very brief, with little or no time for conversation. We acknowledge this reality but still affirm that all interactions can, if we choose, be carried out in a compassionate and sensitive way.

The concept of the three-eye model

This proposed 'three-eye model' was conceived from several different sources. Firstly we drew on our in-depth practical experience of working with groups of health and social care practitioners on the topic of best practice. These groups included nurses, midwives, doctors, social workers, occupational therapists and physiotherapists over many years. Secondly it is based on our personal research interests, and thirdly on several key emerging trends that we identified in the research literature on change.

When we considered best practice and theories of how we change and develop, we noticed markedly different perspectives in the literature. For example, there is a problem-solving, problem-based or problem-focused approach, which we examined in Chapter 2. This approach supports the view that change is largely a problem to be fixed and is best described by a deficit-based theory (Kotter 1998). In marked contrast to this perceived negative and deficit-based approach, we also noted research where change was seen more in terms of opportunity than threat (Jackson & Dutton 1998) and the pioneering work of Cooperrider and Srivastva (1987) and Cooperrider and Whitney (2005). These researchers offer a vision of change that is less problem-focused and more strengths-based. The idea that change emerges from firstly understanding strength, and what is working well, was examined in Chapter 3. In support of this more appreciative view of change, we also noted the emergence of positive psychology and the work of Seligman and Csikszentmihalyi (2000), defined as the scientific study of positive human functioning and flourishing. Seligman (2002) explored what contributes to a fulfilling life well lived and showed how an individual's signature strengths relate to authentic happiness and abundant gratification. Affirming and developing these concepts further has led to the field of positive organisational scholarship, exploring new ways of understanding the processes and dynamics of positive outcomes in organisations (Cameron *et al.* 2003).

When considering these contrasting viewpoints (one negative and driven, the other positive or appreciative and responsive), the temptation is to select one approach as best describing the nature of who we are, and how we change and develop. However, rather than seeking an absolute, we instead need to ask the question: can we offer a more integrated approach and understanding of healthcare education and practice that can accommodate all these perspectives? The 'three-eye model' was conceived and published in response to this question (Machon & Roberts 2010). This particular model, as previously explained, can accommodate both what we call a problem-focused lens (the analytical eye) and an appreciative, more relational perspective (that appreciative eye). In addition, we have considered the value of paradox, as we began to examine in Chapter 4, and how a combined lens (the creative eye) can encompass the best of both, and offer something more than the sum of its parts to the care worker and healthcare practice in general.

Applying the three-eye model in practice

Like any model, the three-eye model represents a map of the territory to be explored. In no way is it intended to describe the full complexity of the human experience. The intention is simply to develop a model that:

- Is as simple and illustrative as possible
- Is integrative, rather than partial or reductive
- Offers insight into the challenges that healthcare practitioners face and illustrates how we can slip into uncaring practice
- Offers the care worker insight and clear developmental steps that can be taken towards sustaining best care practice.

To illustrate how this approach works with clients, and can develop your capacity to care, resourcefulness, emerging skills and qualities as a carer, it is important to consider the application of the 'three eyes' in practice. In this chapter we invite you to think more psychologically about care. We propose that the practice of caring is self-referencing. In other words, the extent of your ability and capacity to care for others directly corresponds to how well you are able to care for yourself. Caring begins with self, and our continual learning and awareness naturally translates to our clients. This means that responsibility for caring rests centrally with the healthcare worker, and as carers we are invited to continually examine our personal and professional development and improvement of practice. It is important to maximise our strengths whilst equally being aware of our edges and vulnerabilities. If conscious and owned, our limitations can actually guide us in how to serve our clients better and offer high-quality safe care.

Pause and reflect

- Are you able to acknowledge your vulnerability and limitations as a care worker as a means of developing a more sustainable healthcare practice?
- What impact does this realisation have on you?
- How can you work with your limitations, rather than against them?

Paradoxically, what can lock and limit our practice is also the key to our liberation and the development of more sustainable practice. Every practitioner should therefore consider their own resourcefulness first and how it is possible to sustain high-quality care. Then consider a further question: what is your most vital resource as a care worker?

Caring – under the spotlight

We rarely consider what defines our resourcefulness as a carer in practice. To do this, the vital resource we are called upon to appreciate and study is our attention. One way of imagining our attention is to think of it as a spotlight that we control. As we concentrate, we can focus its beam. Wherever the beam of light is directed, it illuminates an area that represents our field of conscious awareness. It can be argued that this area marks the extent of the information that our brain can consciously process. The extent of our field of awareness is dependent on our attentiveness. It is therefore central to best care practice to answer the question: how do we learn to concentrate and direct our attention?

Caring at your best

Pause and reflect

- Recall the times when you have demonstrated caring at your very best. What was this experience like?
- What did you notice about your attention?
- Where was your attention?

As researchers, we have asked groups of health and social care practitioners this question in our workshops exploring best practice over many years. Here is a selection of common responses.

What is characteristic of caring at your best?

- I am relaxed and calm.
- I am not feeling under pressure, despite the pressure of work.
- I am interested in my client and wish to really understand them.
- I feel empathy with my client.
- I don't feel the pressure of time and I am not reactive or impulsive.
- I am discovering what my client really wants and needs and the choices they have.
- I am fully engaged with my client.
- I have good trusting rapport with my client.

What do you notice about your attention?
- It is directed towards the client.
- It is given fully to the client.
- It is focused upon the client and I am listening intently.
- I am aware fully of my client and also what's going on for me.

How do these responses relate to your own?

It is interesting to note that people care best when they are able to give their full attention to the client. They experience a relaxed concentration, they are able to listen intently and they have an innate desire to more fully understand the needs of the client.

Caring at your worst

Now let's consider the opposite case – the times when we experience caring at our worst.

Pause and reflect

- What is characteristic of your experience of caring at your worst?
- Where was your attention?

Here is a set of common responses when this question was put to groups of healthcare workers in the same workshops.

What is characteristic of your experience of caring at your worst?
- I am over-busy and don't feel I have time.
- I have too much on.
- I feel anxious.
- I am reactive and impulsive.
- I feel detached and disengaged from my client.
- I'm on autopilot.

Where is your attention now?
- It is all over the place.
- It's dissipated; my light beam is dispersed.
- It's unfocused.
- It is not on my client.
- It is more focused on me.

In this situation, the participants are no longer able to concentrate and focus their attention. They feel anxious, pressured by time and targets, and their field of conscious awareness is greatly reduced and directed more inward, in support of themselves, than outwards to the client and their care needs. They appear to be more in survival/reactive mode than caring mode. The client is likely to be perceived as a problem or threat, rather than an opportunity to care. Thus they find themselves reacting to the needs of the client, rather than being able to offer a caring response.

Such reactions may at best meet the patient's basic care needs – such as handing a client a glass of water (rather than ensuring that water is placed so that they can reach it themselves at all times). But at worst, a negative, reactive view of the client can result in devaluation, overlooking of need, and actual neglect. The current healthcare system often has a very high level of demand and rapid throughput. Not every client requires an attentive and compassionate gaze and relationship, but all care workers should be conscious, open and capable of attuning to those who do require our attention and compassion.

Losing attentiveness – going onto autopilot

Though many of us believe that we can multi-task well, in truth we can pay attention to only one thing at a time. We may learn to quickly switch our attention from one thing to another but we can only do so much multi-tasking before we appear to overload our brains. Our spotlight of attention is distracted and split, and this is why greatly distracted individuals find themselves unable to concentrate and focus.

Under these circumstances, our capacity to understand what is actually happening is greatly diminished. Each and every task, small or large, is experienced as overwhelming and energy depleting. It appears that we have 'outsourced' the ability to manage and control our attention. Instead, our reactions depend on the automatic systems of the brain. When people slip onto autopilot in this way, there can be significant consequences for their behaviour and caring practice. Gaffney (2011, p. 170) notes how 'going on automatic' is often associated with negative feelings and preoccupations and is less optimal working – more 'pretend working'.

Pause and reflect

- For what proportion of your working day do you lose your ability to concentrate and focus your attention?
- When this happens, what do you do about it?
- What is your strategy for refocusing your attention?

Research evidence suggests that we are able to focus and concentrate our attention as little as 5 per cent of the time (Baumeister *et al.* 1998, Muraven *et al.* 1998). This is a surprisingly low figure and offers a stark picture of how frequently we may slip into more automatic, reactive ways of working. Most of us probably assume that this happens much less often than it actually does.

The eye of the autopilot is the first lens we will explore. It is our most habitual way of seeing and it is our default mode. We describe this as 'the unawakened' or 'unconscious' analytical eye. We will explore two forms of the analytical eye: the unawakened and awakened, representing how we use this eye unconsciously and consciously.

The unawakened analytical eye

How it serves

In our evolution as a species, being able to react impulsively, efficiently and practically to an impending physical threat is key to our survival. Baumeister *et al.* (2001) recognises that, in reaction terms, bad is stronger than good. Our attention is grabbed more by negative than positive emotions. Reacting to a physical threat can save our lives but what if the threat we face is less physical and life threatening and more of an emotional challenge – in the form of work pressure? How then does the analytical eye limit our practice?

How it limits

Self-serving

The unawakened analytical eye is less concerned with the needs of others and more with protecting and preserving ourselves. It is defensive and wishes to affirm our sense of rightness through its compulsive problem-solving in order to get to the right answer.

Political

There is little capacity to accommodate the needs of another, and the viewpoint is singular and judged to be absolutely right. This eye is willing to enter into a debate but holds true to its absolute position concerning what it thinks is correct. Through this lens, there is only one way of doing things and that is 'my way'. In this sense, we can view the analytical as a political eye, clear about the importance of our own position and with little or no tendency to accommodate further.

Negative bias and cynicism

The analytical eye develops an automatic preoccupation with the negative – because its vision is primarily problem-centred. This perceived negative bias can become unconscious, and people are unaware of the extent of its influence on their thinking and practice. Langer (2005a, p. 43) highlights the 'tyranny of evaluation' and how this can limit our effectiveness. Through the analytical eye, people may feel compelled to get to the problem and then to rapidly evaluate it, with the intention of fixing or solving it. However, if we only look for problems, that is what we find. This preoccupation with problem-seeking creates a cynical and negative edge to our approach to practice. Through the analytical eye, the care worker may see the client more as a potential threat to well-being than someone to care for. In this sense, the care worker is reacting (rather than responding) to the needs of the client. In all organisations, there is good care practice, but this will go unnoticed by the analytical eye, which is seeking only the problem. We might therefore consider what role the analytical eye plays in creating an insidious negative culture.

Cold, detached and objectifying

The viewpoint of the analytical eye is what we adopt as an external observer. We step outside every situation and, from this detached position, look in and assess objectively. This is experienced as a cold, detached viewpoint. It is by nature a differentiating eye, which is quick to judge this to be right and that to be wrong and intent on identifying difference. It finds the problem and, in so doing, isolates this aspect or part from the whole. In practice, the care worker may see clients objectively, and see them more in part rather than as whole people.

Pause and reflect

You are sitting next to a family member who is in a hospital bed. You overhear a nurse referring to the client in the bed next door not by name but as 'that hip over there in the corner'.

- How does this make you feel?
- Would you do something about it?

This cold, detached objectification is what is seen through the analytical eye and represents a partial sightedness and blindness to the whole person. The unawakened analytical eye can overlook the innate value and humanity of the client and act disrespectfully and in undignified ways. Such actions are central to some of the findings in the Francis Report (2013).

A focus on detail rather than quality

The analytical eye is rational and preoccupied with facts and data. It rapidly focuses on the content and detail and measures success quantitatively and more often by meeting targets and form-filling than by the quality of the care given. In concentrating on the detail, this eye misses the larger context and the opportunity to actively engage the client. It is less interested in asking questions and more in giving answers. The client is then 'dis-engaged' and may be unable to participate in their own care and healing.

A non-empathic approach

By 'standing outside' and looking in objectively, the analytical eye devalues the importance of subjective experience. The care worker is then unable to stand in the shoes of the client and offer an empathic response. Practitioners may turn away from their own inner subjective experiences and compound their fear and anxiety. The analytical eye places little value on what someone is feeling or sensing and is compelled to look at the facts and detailed content of the interaction. This represents a form of emotional avoidance and a tendency to turn away from difficult emotional challenges, both personally and professionally. Not being attuned to the needs of the client, the care worker is likely to equally devalue and overlook their own emotional needs. Lack of self-care of the care worker is a common consequence of the analytical eye. This eye has a limited resourcefulness and quickly becomes depleted and exhausted.

Non-reflective practice

This non-empathic eye is unable to self-reflect. Instantly, everything is judged to be either good or bad, with a resulting impulsive set of action steps. In the compulsion to evaluate, the care worker overlooks the value of being aware of the thoughts and feelings (and indeed the needs) of the client. The care worker then misses the reality of the current moment and what is actually present that they could respond to. Our 'bandwidth of awareness and response' through the analytical eye is very narrow, due to our high degree of preoccupation and distraction. Although we have no doubt about our analysis, all too often we are in error – because we are missing what is actually happening or what is needed by the client. This non-reflective eye lacks the capacity to pace, pause, question and engage. When caught in the analytical eye, it is not uncommon to hear the impatient care worker report that they never have enough time to offer good-quality care. The logic of this eye creates its own mental 'cul de sac', which negates what is ultimately needed – responsive high-quality care.

Reacting to the past, and missing present reality

Absolute information (which we automatically judge to be either right or wrong) is stored directly in our memory. LeDoux (2002) notes that the amygdala is the structure in the brain that is concerned with our reactions to threat. Here, memories are stored as rough, wordless blueprints for emotional life. The price of having a highly reactive amygdala is that negative emotions are easily aroused and we are given to over-reaction. Rather than responding to the present, we react automatically, based on memory and the past. We find ourselves reacting in the same ways we have always reacted, which may not be appropriate for the current situation. Not only may the care worker thus misjudge current need but their response will probably be an over-reaction. This eye will overlook the need to carry out a reality check. It has a form of blindness, an inability to assess what is actually happening here and now. This is in fact a double bind, since when we are caught in the analytical eye we are blind to our own blindness. We are unable to see how we are caught in reaction to, and controlled by, our thoughts and feelings, rather than being able to reflect on and respond to them.

Critical, judgemental, one-dimensional vision
Through the vision of the unawakened analytical eye, we are compelled to evaluate and critically appraise the client situation. This impulse to analyse and evaluate may be turned inward as well as outward. In this way, the care worker commonly becomes the problem and we then judge ourselves harshly. This eye is often plagued with self-doubt and criticism, and appears to account for our neurotic tendencies. The result is that people are often inwardly judgemental of themselves as practitioners and outwardly critical of the client and their needs.

Note how the analytical eye is busy, distracted and self-preoccupied and unable to harness and direct attention towards the client. Attention deficit hyperactivity disorder (ADHD) is a condition where individuals find it a constant challenge to control their attention because it is continually drawn by external distractions and internal negative preoccupations. Interestingly, Hallowell (2005) has noted a growing number of adults with no neurological disorder but who behave with ADHD like symptoms, possessing an attention deficit trait. This is characterised by distractibility, reaction and impatience, an inability to reflect and prioritise and difficulty in managing their time (Hallowell 2005). Fredrickson (2003, p. 166) also noted that, when under threat, people significantly reduce their thought action repertoire and therefore think and act in a very limited, repetitive and uncreative way.

Gilbert and Choden (2014, pp. 38–45) draw a distinction between the 'old brain' and the 'new brain' and their markedly different characteristic behaviours. A central premise is that our 'new brain' capabilities (including our abilities to relate and communicate, imagine, anticipate, reason and plan) can be hijacked by our 'old brain' passions (fear, anxiety and anger), resulting in the experience of feeling threatened and blocked. The grip of the 'old brain' appears to result in the limited vision of the reactive analytical eye. This concept is further described and developed by Peters (2012, pp. 12–19) in considering the 'chimp paradox'. His work highlights how quickly a chimp-like aspect of ourselves can become emotionally driven and threatened, accounting for such behaviours as: jumping to conclusions, 'black and white' thinking and paranoid delusions. Note how these reported observations reflect the limitations of the analytical eye, as described above.

The appreciative eye – key characteristics

We will now look at the influence of the appreciative eye (in contrast to that of the analytical eye) and give you an opportunity to compare your vision of care through each lens.

> 'It is only when we've awakened that we realize how much of our lives we've actually slept through.' *(Langer 2005a, p.16)*

It is critical for care workers to learn how to open the appreciative eye in practice, while they are caught in the unawakened analytical eye. This prospect will be discussed in detail in Chapter 7, where we explore the nature of mindfulness in practice.

How it limits

The lens of the appreciative eye is not content-focused and is therefore unable to ground and contract awareness. Instead, its primary purpose is to expand awareness and one's experience. Structure and focus are considered key to action planning. However, the appreciative eye may be unable to effectively assess, evaluate, prioritise or plan. It can easily generate options but then has no capacity to focus on specific options to inform action planning.

Pause and reflect

Consider how these limitations of the appreciative eye may in fact be complemented by the strengths of analytical eye.

How it serves

Integrative

When we open an appreciative eye, we adopt a different perceptual position – that of the inner observer. This offers the practitioner insight – essentially the capacity to witness, reflect upon, accommodate and respond to subjective experiences. Whereas the analytical eye takes an objective external view, the appreciative eye is both internal and subjective. This experiential eye is able to reflect on our own and our client's inner subjective experience. It is also able to consider the value of what we are actually feeling, thinking and sensing.

This openness to subjective experience may mean that care workers are more flexible and able to accommodate a fuller and more authentic picture of themselves and others. The appreciative eye is therefore a powerfully integrative eye, with a wider bandwidth than the analytical eye. It can significantly expand awareness, helping us overcome the tendency to automatically jump to conclusions, based on partial data and the analytical perspective. In opening the appreciative eye, we become more open-minded. Fredrickson (1998) argues that this open-mindedness and broader mindset offer both indirect and long-term adaptive benefits by building enduring personal resources.

Two-dimensional vision – awareness of self and other

The appreciative eye has a two-dimensional vision, and can therefore accommodate the experiences of both the care worker and the client. Its ability to take several different perspectives and to reflect upon what we, as practitioners, may be feeling, thinking and sensing creates the capacity to attune ourselves to the client's experience – especially their emotional and non-verbal signals. The innate ability to reflect upon emotions means that this eye is unlikely to be overwhelmed by those emotions. In contrast to the analytical eye, the appreciative eye has a natural ability to build rapport with clients and is much more relational.

Empathy

The innate empathic ability of the appreciative eye enables us to become aware of our own subjective experience and that of others. This gives us the capacity to be able to 'stand in the shoes' of the client and to reflect with them about their experience. This capacity allows the care worker to attune to, and be more aware of, the needs and desires of the client. In being able to attune and give our attention to another in this way, we can move beyond evaluation and quieten judgemental and critical activity. Through the appreciative lens, we can build trust by fostering rapport, engagement and personal empowerment. Knowing the facts about why something should be done is essential, but it is emotional awareness that provides the motivation and impetus to change.

Positive bias

With the opening of the appreciative eye, the compulsion to identify and evaluate the problem is potentially stilled. In the absence of this compulsion, there is space for interest and curiosity to motivate a more relational approach. Rather than automatically trying to get to 'the answer', the care worker may begin to seek to question the client more naturally. Once more, this allows the practitioner to build rapport and develop the practitioner–client relationship. It can also foster greater inclusion and shared understanding of what the client ideally wants and ultimately needs. Interest, calmness and curiosity are all qualities that engender a more appreciative and positive approach to client work, and contrast markedly with the negative bias of the analytical eye. Note how being positive and appreciative and feeling happy appears to engender success.

Questioning rather than answering

By no longer feeling compelled to answer, the appreciative lens may motivate practitioners to question the client in a more person-centred manner. Likewise, by being no longer compelled to evaluate, the appreciative eye affords a sense of space and is comfortable with creative uncertainty. Learning how 'not to know' can foster the practitioner's ability to listen more intently and thus respond better to the client's wishes and needs.

Working in the present moment with presence

Since the appreciative eye can self-reflect, it is much better at being present and simply seeing the present reality as it is. This eye thus helps the practitioner make a clearer assessment of the current situation. Being in the present means that individuals are more able to harness and focus their attention intently. The more the care worker is able to give their attention to the client, the more the care worker's presence is felt and experienced by the client.

Pace and pause

The appreciative eye is not busy – unlike the analytical eye. As mentioned earlier, the appreciative eye is therefore comfortable to pause and reflect. This results in the care worker feeling that they have enough time. Having the ability to be still and stop helps the practitioner avoid making premature judgements, since they are no longer compelled to evaluate and rapidly conclude. In this way, the care worker is less distracted and more attentive and able to concentrate on their actual caring role.

Accommodating vulnerability

By reflecting upon subjective experience, practitioners can begin to accommodate both the vulnerabilities and the strengths of the client and indeed themselves and their colleagues. The analytical eye – in rejecting, avoiding and/or denying the value of subjective experience – can create the mask of the perfectionist. It is unable to consider the value of being aware of vulnerability and limitation and simply pretends that the professional role is perfectly right at all times. Below the surface, this can be exhausting for the practitioner. When we ignore our own limitations, we set impossible standards for ourselves and others. In marked contrast, the appreciative eye is able to reflect upon limitation and to consider potential need in relation to vulnerabilities and strengths – both our own as care workers and those of our clients. Through this lens, fears, doubts and anxieties can be acknowledged. In this way, the appreciative eye can tune into the needs of the client and more fully explore their resourcefulness.

To sum up, the appreciative eye is more open and unconditional, and Langer (1997, 2000, 2000a, 2005b) has shown how such an approach results in more engaged effective learning, greater competence and creativity, more positive feelings, less burn-out, better health and even increased charisma.

The potential for synthesis, leading to the creative eye

We have already noted how the limitations of the appreciative lens are balanced by the strengths of the analytical eye. The opposite is equally true and is illustrated in Table 6.1 below (adapted from Machon 2010, p. 47).

Table 6.1: How the limitations of the analytical eye are balanced by the strengths of the appreciative eye

Analytical	Appreciative
Unable to expand awareness	Expands awareness
Grounds/contracts	Unable to ground/contract
Non-reflective	Reflective
Reactive	Able to pace and pause
Non-empathic	Empathic
Able to evaluate and action plan	Unable to evaluate and action plan

Now imagine placing the analytical and appreciative eyes together, as if they were two sides of the same coin. The limitations of one would be precisely cancelled and balanced by the strengths of the other. In combination, a third eye is formed that in prospect offers the strengths of both (see Table 6.2 below) and something more still, as we will now explore.

Table 6.2: The combined strengths of the awakened analytical and appreciative eyes

Self-serving	In service of the other
Objective	Subjective
Contracts awareness	Expands awareness
Reactive	Reflective
Differentiating	Integrating
Isolates the part	Integrates different parts
Non-empathic	Empathic
Answering	Questioning

Pause and reflect

Recall the times when you were practising at your very best.

- What were the characteristic features of this experience?
- What did you experience?
- How were you feeling?
- What were you doing?

The creative eye essentially informs and defines our best practice as care workers and has the following key characteristics.

Developing unconditional positive regard

Whereas the analytical eye is rational and objective, the appreciative eye is subjective and relational, the creative eye (which combines analytical and appreciative aspects) can offer the client what is termed unconditional positive regard. Rogers (1961) credits Standal (1954) with coining the term 'unconditional positive regard'. This describes offering support and acceptance without judgement or conditions, allowing the client to accept themselves and not be caught in others' judgements of their value and worth. In practice we see unconditional positive regard of the creative eye as a modelling of what we paradoxically term 'objective intimacy'.

It is a capacity to be fully present to the client, to attune to them and empathise with them, whilst also having the ability to step back and help the client to process events. Not being over-identified with (or therefore overwhelmed by) the client's experience permits the care worker to remain observant and objective whilst still being empathic and showing understanding. The ability to model respectful detachment, whilst being deeply caring, requires the practitioner to be present and empathic and equally responsive and facilitative. This approach specifically defines how the practitioner serves the client's care. As we will explore further, the capacity to be deeply relational and be motivated by compassion allows the healthcare worker to act at all times with the intention of relieving suffering.

Accommodating present, past and future

In combining and effectively synthesising the appreciative and analytical aspects, the creative lens gains a broad and flexible bandwidth. The care worker who employs a creative lens can help the client to expand their awareness and/or contract it to inform key choices and actions. In this sense, the creative eye is uncompromised. It can concentrate fully, for extended periods of time, and assess current reality and what the present moment requires. It is also comfortable connecting with and recalling past history, as required, and equally able to help set a desired future goal. Through the creative lens, the care worker can see both their own potential and that of the client. They can conceive and facilitate the positive prospect of who the client is aspiring to become. This eye can therefore work totally flexibly and responsively in relation to the past, present and future.

An unlimited eye – uncompromised and responsive

What does the creative eye give us, beyond what is offered by the analytical and appreciative eyes? The simple answer is that it provides the best of both lenses – and something more. Whereas the analytical eye is reactive, and the appreciative eye is relational, the creative eye is responsive and unlimited. This uncompromised and highly flexible lens is able to question and/or help the client to answer; it can focus on context and/or content; it can expand awareness by inviting the client to consider options; and it can contract awareness, helping the client to plan by identifying the next steps they wish to take. This creative lens can view each situation from many different perspectives (appreciative aspect) and can help the client to evaluate, process and action plan (awakened analytical aspect). As we will see in Chapter 8, when we employ the creative lens we can naturally facilitate coaching conversations that foster the engagement of the client in their own care and resourcefulness.

Three-dimensional 'varifocal lens'

The creative eye is rather like a varifocal lens – in that it can be totally flexible and can adapt to, and compensate for, all the limitations of our sight. This reminds us once more of the scope of this lens and how it can accommodate many different perspectives, simultaneously fostering a mental, emotional, physical and spiritual awareness and response. In addition, the creative eye is able to step out and look beyond the individual and relational (the two-dimensional vision of the appreciative eye) to consider how the wider collective (the three-dimensional aspect) can affect an individual. This may allow the care worker to consider, for example, how the organisational culture may be affecting an individual client and respond to the situation.

A motivational eye

The creative eye can be motivational, in that it is able to engage the client's desire and will, and their ability to identify choice and take action. Change is motivated by linking choice with personal values, beliefs and purpose. The creative eye can facilitate this process, thus allowing the client to access and express their personal values, belief and sense of purpose and locate the change they desire. This remembering is equally important for us, as practitioners, enabling us to recognise our values and empowering beliefs and recalling our purpose – why we choose to come to work and do what we do. This sets out a clear intention, as a basis for our commitment to care, and motivates us in our practice.

Through the creative eye, we can truly begin to explore client need. Baumeister (1991, p. 301) notes that this exploration has four dimensions or aspects:

- **Purpose** – believing in something we are moving towards and desire
- **Values** – things we value that make us feel good and positive and help us decide what is right or wrong; goals shaped by values create actions and decisions that have great meaning
- **Self-efficacy** – that we are able to control and manage our attention and make a difference
- **Self-worth** – that we are essentially good and worthwhile.

When these different aspects of need are combined, when client and/or practitioner are clear about their purpose and values and are experiencing personal efficacy and worth, then life and work are experienced as meaningful.

Making meaning

It is important to consider the role of the healthcare worker in helping or enabling the client to make meaning from what is often a challenging situation, as a key step towards engaging their resourcefulness and helping them progress towards well-being. Recall the analytical eye, its reactivity and lack of choice. Seligman and Maier (1967) note how meaningless suffering is the cause of endless human misery, how it steals away our sense of control and blinds our sense of purpose, making us develop a 'learned helplessness'. Making meaning is vital for both care worker and client and holds the key to personal growth.

Csikszentmihalyi (1992) tells us that the meaning of life is making meaning – whatever it is and wherever it comes from. Gazzaninga (1985, 1993) explains how the left hemisphere of our brains interprets and gives meaning to situations by making connections between different aspects, even when there is no actual connection. When a healthcare worker enables a client to make connections and create meaning and discover what choices they have in their situation, it can make a profound difference to the client's sense of control, engagement and motivation. Realising that we have a choice can help us overcome the depressive feeling of helplessness with a positive intent and motivation to make a desired change.

Brickman (1987) explains that 'what we have to do' is very different from 'what we want to do'. The former is negative and enforced; the latter is a choice and potentially liberating. Despite being in crisis, having choices can always be interpreted meaningfully. Note how realising they have choices can transform the client from feeling like a victim of circumstance to feeling more empowered and actively engaged in their care and healing.

Accommodating a spiritual context

The opening of a creative eye offers the care worker and client a further dimension of awareness, recognising our role within the larger whole and instilling a sense of hope in 'something more'. This spiritual context can inform our personal belief system, irrespective of which particular faith we choose to follow. The belief in something 'larger than ourselves' (and realising our connection to, and our place within, this larger whole) can offer an important context for our life and work, potentially bringing great relevance and meaning to challenging situations. Having an awareness of such personal beliefs can positively sustain the practitioner in their professional practice in times of crisis. For the client, recalling empowering beliefs and a sense of purpose can help build resourcefulness and a sense of empowerment despite ill health.

Eliciting resilience and resourcefulness

The creative eye is a resilient eye, in that it can discover opportunity in adversity. Its ability to look at things from many different perspectives allows the care worker to reframe challenging scenarios in such a way as to offer opportunity for the client – for instance, by asking the question: 'Are you learning through your period of ill health?' This may not make the situation easier, but allows the care worker to reframe it in order to invite the client to discover their own choice and resourcefulness as an essential step towards regaining health and well-being. This approach can significantly build resourcefulness and give the client the confidence to make choices and respond positively to adversity.

Working with compassion

When the care worker slips into the creative eye in practice, it allows several unique qualities and capabilities to emerge (beyond the analytical and appreciative ones). One such motive that emerges is the choice to work with compassion. In working with empathy, the care worker becomes attuned to the client's true situation. In addition, through the awakened analytical aspect of the creative eye, they can actively respond. As well as being accepting and empathic, the care worker is able to consciously affirm their motivation to care. When motivated by compassion, our intention is to help relieve suffering. This motivation can be remembered each time we practise consciously building a compassionate perspective on caring.

With dignity

With the opening of the appreciative eye, the care worker can develop a more non-judgemental attitude towards clients and be more wholly accepting of the individual. In experiencing unconditional positive regard, the client can feel safe and trusting and able to explore their own mind, to understand their emotions and potentially feel soothed. In this situation, the client feels met, understood and held and will therefore feel comfortable about sharing and disclosing experiences and feelings.

The creative eye invites the client to be authentic and to work with integrity and to include their vulnerabilities as well as their strengths in exploring how they can fully engage in their treatment programme. In this way, the client's humanity can be acknowledged and affirmed. Practising with dignity involves remembering and respecting the innate value of the client as a human being. This approach supports the creative eye's belief that each individual possesses all the personal resources necessary for their own growth, well-being and fulfilment. The role of the healthcare worker is to see potential and invite resourcefulness in the client, encouraging self-care and initiating positive changes that help to alleviate or end suffering.

When we describe working with the creative eye, people tend to think that keeping up this level of attention must be exhausting. We have found, in practice, that initially consciously adopting this position does take effort. However, in the caring role adopting the creative eye appears to bring great satisfaction and fulfilment. This is because the creative eye is both self-affirming and client-affirming. For example, as we learn to accept and value our own limitations and vulnerabilities, we are equally able to accommodate those of the client. Rather than being exhausting, slipping into the experience of the creative eye therefore often fosters renewed vitality in both carer and client.

Conclusion

This chapter has established the value and potential of the three-eye model. It has illustrated the key characteristics of the analytical, appreciative and creative lenses, and how each of these can affect the care worker's practice. In the next chapter, we explain how the analytical, appreciative and creative eyes inform three markedly different levels of care – namely reactive, relational and responsive. Essentially, we will show how the care worker can, with insight, apply their knowledge of these different levels of care in order to progress towards becoming a compassionate person-centred carer.

Chapter 7

Mindful healthcare practice

Introduction

In this chapter, we explore reactive, relational and responsive caring, as seen through the analytical, appreciative and creative lenses respectively. Reactive caring, as we will see, is a partial and limited, non-person-centred approach. It offers a view of 'shadow' care – less conscious, negative healthcare, including a lack of basic care and, at its most extreme, abusive practices.

Jung (1938) described the 'shadow' as the unknown 'dark side' of our personality. This aspect is 'dark' because it predominantly consists of the primitive, negative, socially or religiously depreciated human emotions and impulses such as hunger for power, selfishness, greed, envy, anger or rage; and, due to its unenlightened nature, it is often completely obscured from our consciousness. In contrast to the 'shadow', we will introduce the concept of mindfulness as it relates to the practice of the care worker. We propose that it is possible to achieve mindfulness through the opening of an appreciative eye in healthcare work practice, leading to a much more relational, person-centred approach to caring. Finally, we will examine the key characteristics and implications of responsive care, and offer guidance as to how the care worker can develop a truly compassionate and person-centred approach to practice.

In Chapter 6, we examined in detail the characteristics of the analytical, appreciative and creative lenses. The vision of each lens offers the healthcare worker markedly different ways of seeing caring practice – namely, reactive, relational and responsive caring. Figure 7.1 (page 72) summarises what defines and differentiates these three approaches to caring.

Reactive care

The drive for efficiency in the NHS, placing more value on targets than clients, can create pressures that make the care worker default to the confined vision of the unawakened analytical eye. Economic and political influences act to speed up, rather than slow down, the care worker in the drive for a competitive edge (Sachs 2011). Such healthcare strategies lock us into our default drive system and we lose sight of the potential damage that we can do under the heading of care.

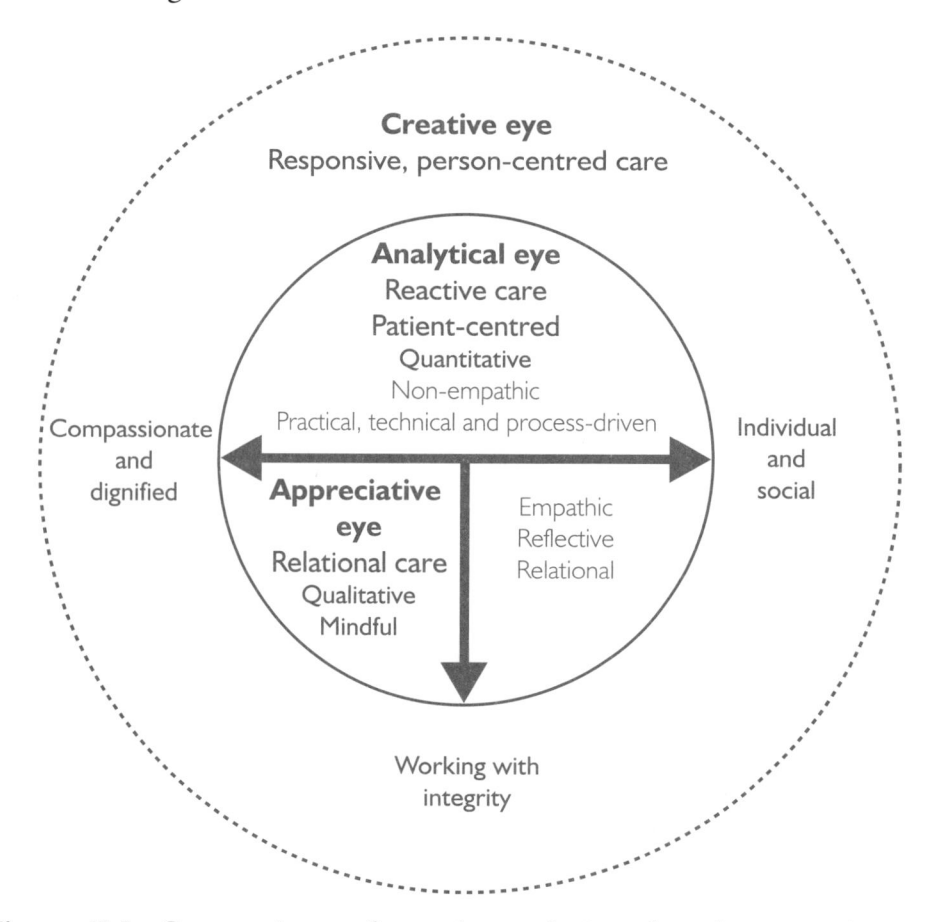

Diagram showing three concentric circles comparing types of care:

- **Creative eye** (outer circle): Responsive, person-centred care
- **Analytical eye** (inner circle): Reactive care, Patient-centred, Quantitative, Non-empathic, Practical, technical and process-driven
- **Appreciative eye**: Relational care, Qualitative, Mindful; Empathic, Reflective, Relational

Surrounding labels: Compassionate and dignified; Individual and social; Working with integrity.

Figure 7.1: Comparison of reactive, relational and responsive care

Gilbert and Choden (2014, p. 74) state very frankly that 'without regulation, either from the outside or within our own moral codes, drives can lead to the worst type of greed and corrupt immoralities, which people will even try to justify'. They go further and say very clearly (p. 75) that 'unregulated drive can promote callousness and indifference towards those who suffer'. If only we could always be aware of the point at which we slip into autopilot, and a driven, reactive attitude to care, it would make it easier to avoid this pitfall. However, as we saw in Chapter 6, the analytical lens is blind to its blindness. This means that when the care worker slips into reactive practice they will rationalise that they are caring perfectly well, whereas in reality they are not. This highlights the vital importance of the three-eye model, which can offer care practitioners the rare opportunity to see and recognise their own blind spots. When they are on autopilot and seeing work as threatening, practitioners are unaware of their negative impact on their clients, and the shadow that they cast in practice.

Features of reactive care

What are the key features that characterise reactive care and what are its implications for the care worker and client?

Self-centred, not client-centred

The care worker is primed to react to potential threats and may commonly see the client through this lens as over-demanding and needy. In this way, the care worker tends to over-estimate the extent of impending danger and negatively over-react. Feeling threatened triggers an age-old, inbuilt 'fight or flight' response in our brains, and this reactive decision is self-centred, rather than being focused on the needs of the client. In essence, the care worker is continually distracted and self-preoccupied.

Non-relational approach

The analytical lens is that of a detached observer and may be experienced by the client as cold and non-relational. When viewing care through the analytical lens, the care worker is unlikely to develop rapport and client engagement beyond a very superficial level. Gilbert and Choden (2014, p. 73) note that 'one consequence of this materialistic self-focus is that it undermines our interests and efforts to build, be part of, and contribute to our social communities'.

Impulsive, problem-focused approach

There is a compulsion to focus on the content, rather than the client. A strong emphasis is placed on client data, instead of the client themselves, and there is an urge to rapidly process and analyse that data, motivated by the impulse to problem-solve and answer questions. Through the analytical lens, the client is commonly perceived as 'a problem' to be fixed. This is a non-person-centred viewpoint that, once more, overlooks the value of actually engaging with the client, and places no value on appreciating client need, knowledge and participation.

Negative bias

The compulsive need to evaluate and the preoccupation of the care worker with problem-seeking and problem-solving results in an approach that the client may commonly experience as negative. In other words, the client is seen as a problem to be critically analysed, judged and assessed.

Answering rather than questioning

Through the analytical lens, the care worker is quick to make absolute black or white assessments and, for example, judge this to be right and that to be wrong. The value of seeking other people's views, including those of the client, is commonly overlooked. The practitioner tends to be directive and to state what the answer is. This negates the value of including the client experience and is marked by a need to answer, rather than engage or meaningfully question.

Objectification

When working through the analytical lens, there is a tendency to objectify the client, whereby the care worker focuses in on a part of the client that is judged to be the problem. In isolating the part, the care worker is unaware of the potential needs of the whole person. This viewpoint is patient-centred and not person-centred. Emphasis is placed on the diagnosis, instead of appreciating or understanding the person. This deconstruction defines the client more as an object than a subject, and may lead the care worker to completely overlook how one part or aspect of the client relates to another. The result is a non-collaborative and differentiated approach to care. Likely consequences include partial diagnosis of the client's condition and care needs.

Content-driven

The analytical care worker is data-driven, preoccupied with content and therefore unable to step back to consider the wider context that informs our reason for caring. Energy is focused on following process and documented practice and making technical and practical interventions. Success, as seen through the analytical eye, is likely to be judged in terms of numbers and targets and administrative form filling, rather than client involvement and satisfaction. Once more the client's experience (what they think, feel, want and need) is undervalued, overlooked and not considered to be a primary concern or even relevant.

A limited view of current reality

The compulsion to analyse, evaluate and process means that the perception of current reality – the actual experience of what is happening here, right now – is at best only partial. Little or no attention may be given to understanding the immediate needs of the client. Instead, client needs tend to be rationalised. What results from such a partial viewpoint is uncaring and, at its most extreme, abusive behaviour.

Not enough time to care

In feeling over-challenged and seeing work as a threat, the care worker may increasingly operate in an impulsive and compulsive way. The ability to reflect, pace and pause is absent, and this may increase the care worker's feeling that they don't have enough time to care. The result may be impatience and potential neglect of clients. The fear of not having enough time, large numbers of clients and the additional preoccupation with meeting objective measures (rather than human need) can quickly build up and overwhelm the care worker. As a result, the carer closes down, becomes distracted and inattentive, and is no longer receptive to client need, centring their energy on coping and survival instead.

In more reflective moments, this protective mechanism leads to guilt, self-reproach and blame, which further diminishes the individual carer's satisfaction with their own performance. Notice the vicious cycle of devaluation: first client, then carer. How can we learn to recognise this cycle and be willing to acknowledge our vulnerabilities and so find the right moment to respond, rather than be caught in reaction? We invite care workers to step forward, voice their concerns and seek appropriate guidance and support through supervision, mentoring and other resources.

Non-empathic invulnerability

The analytical lens, as we have seen, is non-reflective. As a result, it may severely limit the care worker's emotional awareness and intelligence. Facts and data are given priority, while the client's emotions and subjective experience are likely to be overlooked and dismissed, as not adding value. What results is a non-empathic approach to caring. At the heart of this way of seeing is an avoidance of emotions. Hayes *et al.* (2004) examine the nature of emotional avoidance and imply that it is based on the fear that difficult or challenging emotions will be too overwhelming. Over-reaction to and rejection of vulnerability is a likely consequence, and this may lead to the extent of suffering of the care worker and/or client going unseen. It is important to note here that the care worker's inability to own and accommodate their own challenging emotions may also stop them seeing the client's emotions.

It may be equally important to consider whether the care worker's unconscious motivation could be an avoidance of potential inferiority. Gilbert *et al.* (2007) point out that fearful striving to avoid being seen as inferior, or 'not up to the job' is linked to mental health difficulties, especially depression, anxiety and stress. In this avoidance, the individual's humanity – the innate value and respect of the client (and indeed care worker) as a human being – may go unnoticed. The common consequence is an undignified, dispassionate approach to caring that, at its most extreme, may become inhumane. In denying or overlooking vulnerability, the care worker may become trapped behind the mask of a perfectionist. In doing so, the care worker may well set unrealistic expectations and targets for themselves and others. Once more, in not being able to recognise or accept vulnerability, the individual neglects the importance of creating a safe and supportive space for the client to speak openly of their need and vulnerability.

Pause and reflect

If and when you slip into reactive caring mode, consider what the key implications are – for both your client and yourself.

In summary, and with reference to Figure 7.1 (see p. 72), reactive care has a quantitative and dispassionate focus that avoids emotional processing. What energy the care worker has is likely to be expended on the practical, technical and process-driven aspects of caring. There is no natural tendency, through the analytical lens, to build rapport or to actively engage the client as a vital contributor to their own care. The care worker becomes a detached single contributor and unlikely to see the value of a more collaborative approach.

The wider, social aspects of caring are likely to be overlooked and devalued through this lens. The Francis Report (2013) describes how the basic care needs of clients were not met; there was a lack of empathy, compassion and dignity in practice and evidence of non-collaborative working; practitioners were unwilling to take their courage in both hands and speak out about wrongdoing and client abuse. Note how, through the analytical lens, there is potential blindness to, and denial of, a lack of care, with emphasis on more self-centred and self-protective behaviours in practice. It is vital to realise that we can all slip into reactive caring, if we are unable to learn how to manage and direct our attention under pressure. However, with insight, we can lift the veil of denial or avoidance and invite all healthcare workers to become aware of the consequences of reactive caring – namely, disengagement, objectification and lack of empathy for the client as well as an inability to care for themselves.

The degree of detachment inherent in the analytical viewpoint makes one consider the extent of shame and guilt that may be evident and yet denied in the care worker. Gilbert and Choden (2014, p. 144) remind us that 'the problem with shame is that it puts us into hiding not only from others but ourselves. It can be one of the main sources of emotional avoidance: we just don't want to look at the stuff that makes us feel so awful about ourselves'. As we disclose the potential triggers to uncaring practice, we hope we can show equal compassion towards what is being avoided, hidden and denied in the care worker. In Chapter 8, we discuss how, if time is given to the personal as well as clinical perspective, regular supervision with a compassionate orientation can be a vital resource. This type of support enables carers to examine feelings associated with their caring role, including guilt and shame. In this way, self-care and management can help avoid the tendency to reactively place blame elsewhere.

Relational care

Recall for a moment how the strengths of the appreciative lens complement those of the analytical. With this awareness, consider how the key characteristics of caring markedly change when seen through the appreciative lens.

Features of relational care

What are the key features that characterise relational care and what are its implications for the care worker and client?

Being interested and curious to relate

The care worker viewing practice through the appreciative lens is no longer compelled to problem-solve. Impulsiveness and the temptation to reactively evaluate are replaced by a capacity to reflect. Curiosity and a natural interest to explore emerge, together with a more appreciative approach to caring. Having got beyond the automatic compulsion to problem-solve and answer, the care worker can now be more reflective and explore the importance of asking the right question. Becoming a reflective practitioner increases relational capability, thus enabling the care worker to build rapport and client engagement.

Being empathic

What the appreciative lens fundamentally offers the care worker is the capacity to reflect upon and therefore include subjective experience. Through this lens, the care worker is motivated to find out more about the client's subjective experience, how they really are and what they are thinking, feeling and sensing. In being able to attune to and effectively 'step into the shoes' of the client, the care worker gains the ability to model a more empathic approach to caring, and develop and show greater emotional awareness and intelligence.

Qualitative care

The ability to accommodate what the client is subjectively experiencing allows the care worker to develop a much more integrated and complete picture of the client's wishes and needs. Note how relational care is less quantitative and more qualitative – less objective and more subjective. The care worker's vision now becomes two-dimensional, with an expanded relational awareness of both self and other. Through the appreciative lens, the care worker is not likely to objectify and see the client in part. More likely, as a reflective practitioner, they will gain an expanded awareness and experience of the client as a whole person, beyond their clinical diagnosis. In this way, through the appreciative lens, we can aspire to provide truly person-centred care.

The capacity to pace and pause

Moving beyond the compulsive and driven nature of the analytical lens, and becoming an appreciative, reflective practitioner, the care worker develops the capacity to pause, stop, reflect and relate. Despite the pressures of a busy working environment, the care worker now feels under less pressure and therefore feels that they have enough time to care.

Mindfulness in practice

The ability to inwardly reflect, and to explore and consider the value of subjective experience, can offer the care worker a more mindful approach to caring. This enables us to respond, rather than react, to the client. We also essentially learn how to manage our distraction by being able to reclaim, refocus and direct our attention. How this innate ability to step away, and reflect, informs and defines mindfulness in practice will be explored in more detail later in this chapter. For now, it is sufficient to say that more mindful practice allows the care worker to be much more aware and actively in service of the client (as well as themselves). Mindful practice is a vital key that unlocks the prospect of responsive, person-centred care.

A clearer picture of current reality and need
The care worker's capacity to be more reflective and empathic means they are able to extend the bandwidth of their perception and awareness. They can therefore concentrate and focus their attention, producing a more comprehensive and shared understanding of current reality. This results in a clearer and more accurate picture and appreciation of the immediate needs of the client.

Accepting both strength and vulnerability
Approaching caring with a more open mind and heart, and building an expanded awareness that includes the client's subjective experience, enables the care worker to explore the strengths and positive attributes the client may wish to employ in their own care programme. Such openness also allows the care worker to listen to what the client wishes to share, concerning their fears and vulnerability. Gilbert and Choden (2014, p. 174) highlight the importance of this process of 'descent' and describe it as 'a willingness to drop down in the unpredictable messy humanity that we normally prefer to sanitise and avoid'.

Once more, it is important to emphasise that the care worker's capacity to be emotionally aware and intelligent applies to their ability to process and accommodate both the client's emotions and their own. One informs the other. What motivates the care worker to be able to work in this way is a compassionate orientation to care. We are reminded that 'the call of compassion is the courage to make the descent in a compassionate way, neither rationalising nor getting overwhelmed and turning away'.

Pause and reflect
If and when you slip into relational caring, consider what the key implications are – both for your client and yourself.

In summary, relational care is markedly different from reactive care. The care worker develops relational competencies through their capacity to be a reflective practitioner. The result is the building of rapport and engagement, motivated by an interest and curiosity to know. Having gained greater awareness of the client's present needs, the care worker can quite naturally explore with the client how they feel and what they desire.

Responsive care

We will now consider the third level of care – the result of seeing caring through a creative lens. First, let us recall how the creative eye combines the strengths of both the analytical and appreciative lenses, whilst negating their limitations, and how this influences and develops the practitioner's capacity to care.

Features of responsive care

What are the key features that characterise responsive care and what are its implications for the care worker and client?

A compassionate motivation to care

The creative lens marries the empathic element of the appreciative eye with the practical element of the analytical eye, enabling the client to process, evaluate and action plan. Note that the analytical element is no longer unconscious and reactive but can now be employed responsively, depending on need. This combination motivates the practitioner to work with compassion. In combining empathy with an intention to act in service of the client, the care worker can access what we call 'an objective intimacy'. On the one hand, the care worker is deeply empathic and can explore the needs and desires of the client, and on the other they are able to retain an element of objectivity in order to act to relieve suffering. This ensures a deeply caring and compassionate approach in practice and at the same time prevents the care worker from becoming overly attached or developing an unhealthy dependency.

Accepting and non-judgemental

In viewing care work through the creative lens, the practitioner develops the capacity to give their full attention to the client. Impulsivity to act ends and the care worker is able to be much more attentive and alert. A marker of such an approach is the development of an unconditional positive regard, meaning that the care worker practises being accepting and non-judgemental. This capability further extends their bandwidth of awareness and perception, allowing them to be highly attentive and able to listen more intently. The client, in turn, experiences the care worker's more attentive presence and feels more fully seen and heard. In these periods of interaction, there is a deepening sense of trust and safety that gives the client the opportunity to be open, honest and willing to disclose and share.

Focused on the client's needs and desires

The creative care worker is more responsive and develops a relaxed and alert concentration. This ability to concentrate, and focus attention on the client, allows the care worker to assess the client's current reality and present needs and desires more fully.

Flexibility and responsiveness
What results from seeing caring through the creative eye is a flexible response, mindful of the needs and desires of the client. Important information from the past may then be offered by the client, together with absolute clarity about their current situation and a shared understanding of desired future outcomes for treatment and care. This lens can therefore be both flexible and responsive in terms of offering both qualitative and quantitative care, depending on the client's requirements. The care worker can concentrate more fully and work more deeply with the client.

Engaging the client's resourcefulness
In Chapter 8, we will explore the nature of the coaching conversation and how this is essential to responsive caring. Here, it is sufficient to acknowledge how the care worker, through the vision of the creative lens, can help the client identify clear goals and explore how these align with their core values and beliefs. Aligning desired goals with values, needs and wishes enables the client to be more resourceful in times of challenge. Conversations that engage and empower the client to consider what resources they can bring to their own care may also help them work towards well-being, health and healing. Discovering choices and opportunities in times of adversity is the means by which the client recognises and builds resilience.

Social awareness
In responsive caring, the practitioner can add a social dimension to their awareness and work. In effect, this means that they develop a social conscience that includes, and is able to look beyond, the immediate needs of the individual client in order to consider wider social implications. For example, the creative care worker will naturally examine any wider social considerations that could affect the care of the client, whether positively or negatively. Such social awareness ensures that a collaborative team approach is applied to client care. This in turn supports a more integrated approach to clinical diagnosis and treatment, and a more widely supported care programme that integrates personal, interpersonal and wider aspects of social care.

Person-centred care
The practitioner is now able to see the client as a whole person and to consider all their physical, psychological, emotional, spiritual, behavioural, environmental, occupational and social needs. This vision allows them to practise truly person-centred care. This is a much more integrated and inclusive approach and places the central value on the client, modelling dignity in practice.

Self-care
The creative eye not only accommodates the needs, desires, wishes and choices of the client but also those of the care worker. This means that the care worker is equally aware

of their own resilience and resourcefulness. Responsive caring essentially starts with the care worker and then naturally extends to the client and others. It acknowledges that the care worker is responsible for managing their own resourcefulness and capacity to care. We need to be clear about our own strengths, motivation, sense of purpose and the values that we bring to work, and be in service of self as well as other. In view of the pressures of life for a healthcare worker in today's NHS, it is vital to be a reflective practitioner and maintain a conscious work–life balance in order to sustain healthy best practice.

Time should be continually dedicated to exploring the challenges of practice and the resources needed (both personal and organisational) to support and sustain a compassionate approach to person-centred care. The care worker will benefit from individual and group supervision, where their learning edges as a care practitioner can be safely discussed in support of continual learning and development. In supervision, strengths and resourcefulness can be explored, together with limitations and vulnerabilities, to enable the practitioner to learn how to achieve health and social care best practice. The value of supervision in this context will be more fully explored in Chapter 8.

Pause and reflect

If and when you slip into responsive caring, consider what the key implications are – both for your client and yourself.

To recap, in responsive caring the client is seen as a vital and equal partner and is actively engaged in defining, agreeing and implementing care. The insightfulness of the creative lens reminds us of a belief that lies at the heart of care work: not only does the client hold answers that are key to their care and well-being but by expressing their desired goals in line with their personal values, beliefs and purpose the client can ignite their own resourcefulness and resilience, which may be vital to their healing.

The creative care worker demonstrates a non-judgemental acceptance of the client that allows them to offer compassionate and dignified care. When met with the negativity of suffering, the care worker does not recoil but offers the positivity of acceptance and a concern to respond. As Fredrickson (2003) notes, compassion does not 'just sit there'; it motivates action to relieve suffering. The analytical aspect of the creative lens is evident and can be employed at any time in processing and action planning, for example. The practitioner is now able to work extremely flexibly and authentically, offering qualitative and quantitative aspects of care, as required. At the same time, the care worker develops a social conscience and awareness that allows for a more collaborative approach to person-centred care.

Becoming a responsive, person-centred carer

As we have seen, the creative lens accommodates the emotional awareness and intelligence of the appreciative aspect, whilst also offering an expanded social awareness. The care worker is now able to quite naturally include the experience of the client as essential to their care programme. In responsive, person-centred healthcare, the client is empowered as a vital active participant in the design and implementation of their own care.

The person-centered approach is increasingly recognised as a gold standard in care practice. In the UK, it is built into the National Health Service Frameworks, monitoring requirements and legislation. For example, the NHS Constitution (NHS 2013, p. 3) has person-centred care as one of its seven core principles, stating that 'the NHS aspires to put patients at the heart of everything it does'. It goes on to describe how NHS services must reflect, and should be coordinated around and tailored to, the needs and preferences of patients, their families and other carers. The need to include and consult patients, their families and carers is clearly affirmed.

Starfield (2011) distinguishes between person-centred and patient-centred (or client-centred) care. When we see an individual as a patient, rather than a person, we focus only on the particular diagnosis (remember the analytical eye's tendency to objectify). Patient-centred (or client-centred) care is therefore only likely to partially meet the client's needs. Bechtel and Ness (2010) highlight five key aspects of care:

- 'Whole-person' care
- Coordination and communication
- Patient support and empowerment
- Ready access
- Autonomy.

Note the value of the care worker's appreciation of the client's life situation, home environment, personal preferences, experiences and care-giver status. As a result, care is more realistic, closely aligned with the client's values and likely to engage the client more fully. Working in partnership with the client tends to lead to more effective health decisions based on complete and unbiased information when assessing, for example, a range of treatment options and/or reviewing side effects and risks and benefits.

The creative lens of the care worker fosters co-creation. The care worker demonstrates trust and respect, compassion and dignity, qualities that are the foundation of responsive, person-centred care. In this way, meaningful relationships are co-created, which are genuine partnerships built upon effective communication (another of the 6 Cs). Responsive, person-centred care naturally includes an emphasis on collaborative working (recall the social awareness of the creative lens). The responsive care worker therefore ensures that healthcare services are working together to deliver care that is mindful of individual needs and abilities, preferences, lifestyles and personal goals. This offers a key element of control and empowerment back to the client, their family and wider network in order to promote independence and full engagement in their treatment and healing process.

The mindful care worker

When caring through the analytical lens, no space exists between our thoughts, feelings and actions. The result is impulsive action, where our thoughts and feelings dictate our reactions. According to Gilbert and Choden (2014, p. 73), this 'striving, getting, having, achieving and owning is almost like an addiction'. Pani (2000) believes this compulsive activity is a consequence of over-stimulation of our dopamine receptors and our sympathetic nervous systems. In contrast, the appreciative healthcare practitioner learns how to be more reflective. Without space for reflection – a chance to pause – work can become exhausting. If pace and the ability to pause are absent from our daily work, we lose our balance. The analytical lens does not punctuate time with pauses or full stops. It is only when we learn how to reflect that we are able to notice and foster a sensitivity to what we are thinking and feeling.

The capacity to pause is the hallmark of the reflective and appreciative practitioner. In learning to reflect upon thought and feeling, we discover that we can choose to respond rather than react. This is a vital shift. Stepping back and reflecting minimises distraction and allows us to reclaim our lost attention and then more consciously deploy this vital resource. This capacity permits us to expand our field of conscious awareness and become open-minded rather than closed. The key question is: how do we learn to activate this vital switch that will expand our vision beyond the analytical, and thus enable us to become more relational and responsive carers? Here is a short activity that may help you achieve this transition.

A short introductory exercise in mindfulness

- Whilst reading this page, we invite you to simply become aware of your breathing...
- Focus your attention on your breath and begin to notice the natural rhythm of your in-breath and out-breath. Pause from reading for a moment and count your breaths. Notice the natural rhythm of your breathing...
- As we guide you through this brief exercise, step by step, see if you can remain aware of your breathing throughout.
- If your mind attempts to take your attention away and starts to analyse and process, simply focus your attention back on your breath. This is quite natural.

- Now we invite you to turn your attention inward and look in at your thoughts. Ask yourself 'What am I thinking?' whilst remaining aware of your breath…
- Take your time to simply notice what you are thinking…
- If you slip into processing or analysing your thoughts, don't worry. Just bring your attention back to watching your breath and then, once again, look in at your thoughts and notice what you are thinking…
- Then ask yourself 'What am I feeling?' And in the same way as you watched your thoughts, simply notice your feelings, whilst staying aware of your breathing.
- Again, analysis is not necessary. Just watch and notice your feelings…
- Now become aware of your physical body and ask yourself 'What am I sensing?'
- Once again, notice what you are sensing in your body. Simply sense your body, whilst staying conscious of your breathing – the in-breath and the out-breath…
- Then bring your attention to your feet placed on the ground, and your body in your chair. Now bring your attention fully back into the room and to what you are reading.
- 'Welcome back'.

Pause and reflect

- What was your experience of this mindfulness exercise?
- How are you feeling now?
- What did you do in this exercise?
- How might this exercise be valuable to your practice?

Following this brief exercise, care workers in our workshops commonly report feeling more calm and relaxed. If you found it a challenge to keep your attention focused, then bear in mind that this is commonly the case and the invitation is simply to keep bringing your attention back to your breathing. Notice how the resulting calmness contrasts with the feelings of stress, anxiety and fear that are commonly associated with the analytical eye. The compulsion to 'do' is somehow dissipated. How does this happen?

To achieve this shift in experience, you simply changed perspective or moved your perceptual position. Though it may sound strange, what you did was to turn yourself inside out – in a very positive way! You turned your attention inward rather than outward. You took the position of being an inner witness and started to reflect on your subjective experience. In watching your breathing, you are using your breath as a focal point and so you are able to reclaim and concentrate your attention. When drawing your attention to this point, note how you indirectly let go of your compulsion to analyse and, as a result, your mind is able to be still and quiet.

If you repeatedly practise this short activity, you will find that you are no longer just reacting to your thoughts and feelings. Instead, you will be able to witness and observe them. If you think of your work as being like a very long unpunctuated sentence, mindfulness practice enables you to add commas and full stops to make more sense of the words. What we do in these pauses is to look at and reflect upon our inner experiences. We are then able to explore and accommodate that which we previously reacted to. Hasson (2013, p. 68) notes that 'accepting the emotion simply means letting the emotion be there, without trying to change the feeling, the experience or the event that prompted it'. Furthermore, observing and accepting (rather than reacting to) what we are feeling relieves us of needless extra suffering.

The nature of mindfulness

Siegel (2007, p. 5) views mindfulness as 'a waking up from life on automatic'. This definition is useful, since it reminds us of the automatic and impulsive nature of the analytical lens to which we default when we feel under threat. In becoming more reflective, the care worker can open an appreciative eye, marking a distinctive shift in our vision and experience of caring. Mindfulness allows the care worker to literally awaken to becoming a more reflective and relational carer. The mindful care worker develops a more open mind and no longer feels compelled to evaluate and analyse.

Langer (1989) reminds us that one of the simplest and most natural methods of reducing self-evaluation is to assume a mindset of mindfulness rather than mindlessness. Through mindfulness practice, we gain the ability to quiet and still our minds, ultimately ending impulsivity by silencing the voice of the inner critic and judge. According to Kabat-Zinn (1994), this does not mean that you cannot make judgements. Rather, it means ending the tendency to constantly judge ourselves in a critical light, which is an insatiable form of irrational tyranny (Williams *et al.* 2007).

Pause and reflect

Imagine, for a moment, what it would feel like to be conscious but without a busy mind or an active inner critic – to have a mind free of noise or activity, with no inclination to judge.

- What does this state of mind offer you?

Mindfulness is the capacity to be attentive and aware without the compulsion to analyse or solve. What develops from this is the capacity to be present and attentive without distraction. We become fully alert, yet relaxed and reflective, and we are able to consciously respond to our thoughts and feelings. We can then cultivate a moment-to-moment non-judgemental awareness (Weick & Putnam 2006). Kabat-Zinn (1994, p. 180) defines mindfulness as 'the awareness that emerges through paying attention on purpose, in the present moment, and non-judgementally to the unfolding of experience moment by moment'. According to Gilbert and Choden (2014, p. 135), mindfulness stops the problems of:

- Attention hopping – the butterfly mind hopping from one thing to the next
- Rumination and brooding – the tendency to turn things over and over negatively in our minds
- Emotional avoidance – blocking out emotions that we deem to be unwanted and painful.

When the care worker is able to cultivate a non-judgemental attitude, they can give the client their unconditional positive regard. This is a capacity to accept unconditionally, without the compulsion to judge critically. If we can stop identifying with our thoughts and simply witness them, then we can discover a new sensitivity to what we are actually thinking. In being mindful, we create a vital space to observe and discover more about ourselves. The UK Mental Health Foundation's report on Mindfulness (Mental Health Foundation 2010) bears this out, and states that this practice can help the healthcare worker to become more aware of their thoughts and feelings, less enmeshed in them and more able to manage and accommodate them.

Consider how mindfulness can allow us to see the reality of the present moment more clearly and thus become better able to assess the immediate needs of our clients. Dane (2011) also reminds us that mindfulness is a state of consciousness in which attention is focused on present-moment phenomena occurring both externally and internally. Note that whatever we experience internally has an external consequence. When you are able to stand apart and simply observe your thoughts and feelings, you simultaneously become able to attune to the thoughts and feelings of others. Mindfulness informs the ability of the care worker to relate to others. Through mindfulness practice, we as care workers can learn how to expand the bandwidth of our conscious awareness, developing insight into our own experience and that of others and so becoming able to notice things more incisively.

Ultimately, we can gain a clearer and more complete picture of the client's immediate and future needs, as well as a growing awareness of our own needs. In this way, we cultivate a capacity for metacognition (Allen & Hancock 2008), an ability to reflect on our own experience, the client's experience and our shared experience. This expansion of emotional awareness and the capacity to process emotions means we are no longer likely to feel overwhelmed. Instead, we can develop an emotional awareness and intelligence in client relationships. As care workers, we are less likely to be distracted by detailed content and more likely to see the overall context of our work and to be able to act with this awareness.

Through mindfulness practice, we become curious to discover more about our clients and indeed ourselves. In our willingness to share experiences, we allow the client to include and integrate their thoughts and feelings. This helps us to create a much broader picture and shared reality and to agree on the most authentic, effective response to their needs.

To conclude, let's summarise the potential benefits of mindfulness for the care worker. Langer (1989, 1997, 2000, 2005b) notes how mindfulness allows us to actively keep our minds open to the novelty and uncertainty in all situations, rather than developing a fixed view. Through this open-mindedness, the care worker is able to engage with clients, learn effectively, achieve greater competence, experience more positive feelings, demonstrate creativity, experience less work burn-out, and gain better health and even increased charisma. Chaskalson (2011) summarises a plethora of published studies showing that there is growing evidence that mindfulness is effective in:

- Reducing stress and increasing emotional intelligence
- Raising awareness of self and others
- Increasing interpersonal sensitivity and communication skills
- Lowering rates of health-related absenteeism
- Increasing concentration and extending attention span
- Reducing impulsivity
- Improving the capacity to retain and manipulate information
- Lowering levels of psychological distress and elevating levels of well-being and life satisfaction.

Conclusion

We have explored and compared the nature of reactive, relational and responsive care, as envisioned through the analytical, appreciative and creative lenses respectively. Rather than consider these as three distinct modes of caring, it may be more useful to see them as a continuum, ranging from uncaring to responsive person-centred care.

In practising the opening and applying of a creative lens, the capacity to care becomes more person-centred. The care worker becomes both relational and responsive, enabling the client's desired choices to be more fully defined and included as central to their well-being and potential healing. The motivation and resourcefulness of the client are engaged to act and participate in their own care and to bring about desired changes that may assist their healing. Note also how the creative lens expands awareness beyond self and other to accommodate a wider social dimension. This ensures a more collaborative and integrated approach to client care.

We have explored how the initial opening of the appreciative eye is a vital step in awakening to reflective practice and empathic care and that mindfulness in daily practice allows the practitioner to operate this essential on-switch to relational care. This chapter has highlighted the essential role of mindful healthcare practice in developing responsive, compassionate person-centred care.

In summary, mindfulness offers the care worker:

- A capacity to reflect upon self and other/client
- A deeper emotional awareness and intelligence that accommodates vulnerability as well as strengths of self and other
- An ability to see beyond the diagnosis and view the client as a whole person
- A capacity to engage the client's resourcefulness and motivation, enabling active participation in their own care programme and the development of self-care and potential healing
- A social awareness that ensures a more collaborative approach, naturally engaging with co-workers, multi-disciplinary teams and the support of extended carers.

In Chapter 8, we will explore what it means to be an appreciative and creative practitioner. We will also explain how the care worker can enable the client to take positive steps towards realising and employing their best and most resourceful self in their care programme. The essential role of the coaching conversation will be highlighted and illustrated as the means by which the practitioner can elicit the client's resourcefulness and their motivation to make positive change.

Chapter 8

The appreciative care worker and coach

Introduction

This chapter highlights the vital role of the coaching conversation in compassionate, person-centred care and how, in becoming a more appreciative practitioner, the care worker develops an approach to caring that naturally facilitates their capacity to coach. We will explore what defines the coaching conversation and its particular structure, and how this type of interaction enables the client, in times of ill health and adversity, to engage more fully in self-care and to recognise their own resourcefulness and resilience.

In addition, this chapter will focus on the essential qualities and skills of the appreciative healthcare worker and coach. We will also demonstrate why the supervisory role should be expanded to support the continual development of care workers' coaching capabilities as well as their clinical and technical competencies. Supervision can then become a vital and trusted individual and group resource for the care worker to develop both personal and professional skills in order to sustain their daily practice of compassionate, person-centred care.

What does it mean to become an appreciative practitioner?

When the healthcare worker is able to employ an appreciative lens more consciously, a major shift occurs in practice and the attitude to caring changes. Rather than being self-concerned and problem- or threat-focused, the care worker becomes much more relational, client-aware and person-centred. When caught in the unawakened analytical eye, we are prone to reactively experience work as a threat, problem-seek and critically judge. The result is a more negative and cynical view of work and indeed caring. Note that when the appreciative eye is opened, we essentially move from being detached, objective and non-relational to becoming more reflective and relational practitioners. As we develop reflective practice, the impulse to problem-solve is replaced by the capacity to pace and pause. The compulsion to react and drive forward is replaced with a growing patience, curiosity and a desire to reflect. Awareness can then expand, resulting in a deeper appreciation and understanding of the wishes and needs of both care worker and client. The care worker becomes less anxious and distracted, and more relaxed and attentive.

Pause and reflect

Recall an occasion when you have been more reflective and appreciative in your work.

- What did this give you as a care worker?

In a nutshell, when the impulse to react and find the answer is no longer present, the care worker discovers a quieter, more open mind. The capacity to 'not know' may bring a new sense of spaciousness and calm. This ability to be more relaxed and alert is a consequence of the care worker being able to refocus and reclaim their attention. In effect, the care worker becomes much less distracted and much more attentive. Rather than directing their attention outward (in seeking to answer and problem-solve), they can now redirect it inward, developing new insight and awareness by exploring and potentially accommodating their own and indeed the client's subjective experience.

The appreciative care worker becomes much more aware of what they are feeling, thinking and sensing. Gilbert and Choden (2014, p. 108) see this as 'a capacity to be sensitive with open awareness' and argue that, with this sensitivity, we are 'less likely to turn a blind eye or use denial or justification to avoid engaging with things we find painful'. This is in marked contrast to the unawakened analytical lens, through which we react to what we are thinking, feeling and sensing, which commonly leads to emotional avoidance or denial. Consider the impact of moving from an objective to a more subjective way of working. By becoming appreciative practitioners, we can expand our awareness of both self and other, and find a new motivation to relate, and a natural curiosity to understand what the client may be feeling, thinking and sensing.

The potential result is a clearer awareness and appreciation of the client's desires and needs, two aspects that are essential to developing a more caring practice. Through the appreciative lens, we can develop the vision to see beyond objective superficiality and to become much more aware of the potential for positive engagement and change. In becoming aware of the client's needs and the changes they would like to make, we can harness the client's intention and motivation to bring about positive change, irrespective of the difficult circumstances they may face.

The appreciative care worker thus becomes aware of a positive potential in the client (and indeed themselves) that is a source of motivation. This can offer a vital sense of direction and choice in times of challenge, which can bring about positive engagement and change that could be vital to the client's well-being. Fredrickson (2001) affirms that a positive and appreciative attitude, which puts us in touch with our desire to bring about positive change, expands our capacity for more creative and innovative thinking, whilst fostering well-being. Note also, as a care worker, that such an appreciative approach appears to be contagious and seems to result in upward spirals of positive practice. In this way, appreciative practice can inspire others and therefore positively influence and inform organisational culture.

Pause and reflect

Think about how appreciative practice can assist positive changes in the culture of the organisation you work for.

Summarise the marked changes that occur when you become an appreciative care worker – for example, gaining a positive approach to your work that fosters rapport, engagement and relationship; finding comfort in working with subjective experience, including both strengths and vulnerabilities; and recognising the need that empowers the client to make positive choices in support of their self-care whilst also potentially bringing about positive individual and cultural change.

Another major aspect of becoming an appreciative practitioner is acknowledging how we can learn how to change from being reactive and threat-driven to being more emotionally aware, affiliative and self-soothing. According to Gilbert and Choden (2014, p. 92), the 'important role of the soothing/affiliation system is to regulate threat-based emotions and bring us back into balance'. In addition to rediscovering a source of motivation and a clearer intention for both the client and care worker, this expansion of awareness facilitates the discovery of a more authentic and resourceful self. By identifying clients' needs and their conscious desire to change, and translating desired goals into personal choices and actions, the care worker can help the client to recognise their own resourcefulness at times of challenge, thus building their resilience, empowerment and confidence.

Developing resourcefulness and authenticity

The pioneering coaching work of Gallwey (2000) offers the healthcare worker insight into how to be more resourceful and authentic, by becoming aware of two key aspects of the self, which he named 'self-1' and 'self-2'.

He described self-1 as our critical, judgemental and often self-condemning aspect, a know-it-all who mistrusts and so impedes the innate and natural ability of self-2. In its critical judgements and reductive and partial thinking, self-1 undermines our sense of wholeness, autonomy and adequacy.

In contrast, self-2 represents our most able self – the person we most desire to become. Gallwey (2000, p. 7) notes that 'self-2 embodies all the inherent potential that we were born with, including all the potential capacities we can actualise and one's innate ability to learn and grow'.

Marrying Gallwey's work with our three-eye model, self-1 represents the way we view ourselves through the lens of the unawakened analytical eye. Self-2, on the other hand, represents a more complete human being (the person we are when we are at our most able, authentic and resourceful) and constitutes the vision seen through the creative lens. The golden question for the care worker, mindful of the grip of self-1, is: how do we remember and learn how to access more of self-2? Gallwey (2000, p. 29) offers the care worker and coach wise guidance: 'we need to learn how to distract or quieten self-1, in order that self-2 can be more fully expressed'.

How do we learn to draw attention from self-1 in order to more fully recognise and realise the potential of self-2? This question is answered in detail in Chapter 7. As we have seen, mindfulness practice offers us the means to go beyond impulsiveness by developing the reflective capacity to witness and observe thoughts and feelings, rather than reacting to and avoiding them. Instead of being controlled by our subjective experiences, we can (through mindfulness practice) learn how to watch and accommodate our thoughts and thus stop being driven by them. In drawing attention to the inner observer, we indirectly distract attention from self-1. As a result, the inner voice of self-1 can be quietened, and the qualities and capabilities of self-2 can then naturally emerge in the presence and practice of the healthcare worker. As Gallwey (2000, p. 12) reminds us: 'paradoxically it is the conscious acceptance of oneself and one's actions as they are that frees up both the incentive and capacity for spontaneous change'. Downey (2003, p. 46) also advises us to open up to the experience and capability of self-2, when 'the practitioner is focused, relaxed and trusting'.

In conclusion, in opening the appreciative eye, the care worker is able to work more mindfully, which facilitates the emergence of their natural ability to reflect and relate. By opening the creative eye, they then naturally become a more resourceful, authentic and able caring worker. This particular transition, from a threat-driven to a more relational and affiliative stance on care, dramatically changes the care worker's attitude and approach and therefore also the nature and structure of their conversations with the client. Rather than telling the client what to do, the care worker is able to engage and question them, appreciate and understand their needs, and help them to be empowered to respond. The nature and structure of the coaching conversation will now be illustrated.

The care worker as coach

What is coaching?

Here are three definitions of coaching:

- 'The role of the coach is to increase choices [of the client]' *(Dembkowski et al. 2006, p.10)*
- '[Coaching is] a drawing out of people's strengths, helping them to bypass personal barriers and limits in order to reach their personal best' *(Dilts 2003, p. xiii)*
- '[Coaching involves] unlocking a person's potential by helping them to learn rather than teaching them' *(Whitmore 2004, p. 8)*.

Incorporating these ideas, we believe the role of the care worker coach is to view the client as able, resourceful, creative and whole, eliciting their resourcefulness and potential by empowering them to make the changes they desire that will relieve their suffering and foster their well-being and health.

This role can be realised in practice through the coaching conversation. What makes the coaching conversation different from any other conversation? Firstly, the care worker sees the client as holding information and knowledge that is key to their well-being and potential health. Despite being an expert and having technical knowledge that is important to the client's treatment, the care worker coach consciously places the client in the 'driving seat', recognising that the client holds vital information concerning their own care, well-being and growth. Acknowledging such value in the client maintains respect and dignity. In adopting a coaching approach, the care worker is non-directive and seeks to empower and engage the client as a vital part of their own care. The approach is fundamentally relational and invites the client to express, and is appreciative of, their desired needs and outcomes. Coaching presupposes that the client alone has the answers needed for their care and well-being.

How can the three-eye model enable coaching?

We have seen that a key first step to becoming a healthcare worker and coach is to open a more appreciative eye in practice. The care worker discovers the means by which they can reclaim their attention and give it more fully to the client. As the alert attentiveness of the care worker develops, the creative eye opens and key aspects of the appreciative and analytical eyes consciously combine to create the basic aspects of the coaching conversation.

The creative eye encompasses both the appreciative element (the care worker's ability to reflect and to relate) and the awakened analytical element (their capacity to facilitate processing of information and action planning, helping the client to define their key next steps). When practising the use of a creative lens, the appreciative healthcare worker may discover that they are able:

- To demonstrate flexibility in being able to both expand and contract client awareness
- To be more fully present in the moment
- To show acceptance and non-judgement
- To be able to question rather than answer
- To look beyond the client's detailed content and consider the context of the work
- To be emotionally aware and empathic
- To be able to work with client values, beliefs and passion
- To demonstrate compassion, in being mindful to act at all times to relieve suffering.

The structure of the coaching conversation

How do these emerging skills and qualities of the appreciative healthcare practitioner enable coaching? There are a number of models that illustrate the coaching process.

The one we offer has the acronym CARE to help identify and remember the four key steps to be followed in the coaching conversation:

- **Step 1** – Compassionate orientation
- **Step 2** – Allow the client to share their goal and desired outcome
- **Step 3** – Reflect on current situation and possibilities
- **Step 4** – Empower and enable the client to take action

Coaching is a way of helping the client rediscover their inner compass, which gives them a strong sense of direction and a motivation to change, by aligning with their goals, desired outcomes and choices. It is the care worker coach's role to help the client set these vital compass bearings and be resourceful. The four key steps of the coaching conversation will now be expanded and studied in more detail.

Step 1 – Compassionate orientation

This first step invites the care worker to consciously take on a compassionate approach to the client. As we have seen, it is all too easy to slip into habits of uncaring practice – for example, by simply responding and reacting to the pressures of work. Therefore, the first step in coaching is to remember the motivation to coach and care. When caught in the unawakened analytical eye, the motive is one of self-protection and self-preservation, whereby the care worker reacts to work more as a threat than an opportunity to care. Through simple mindfulness exercises and practice, we can learn to see how we are caught in reaction and instead to acknowledge what we are feeling and thinking. This enables us to step away from the reflex of reacting to, and avoiding, subjective experiences. We can also learn to step out of negative ways of working and to concentrate and consciously affirm the value of an appreciative approach to caring.

As a first step, we need to remember our reason for choosing healthcare work and our motivation to be a compassionate, person-centred care worker. Gilbert and Choden (2014, p. 48) remind us that compassion is a 'social mentality', since it is 'focussed not just on self but also on one's interaction with others and how we respond to the ways that they interact with and react to us'. Taking a compassionate orientation means that the client is not seen as a threat or challenge but instead respected as a vital and valued resource, whose desired goals and outcomes are key to their care and well-being. This compassionate approach views the client as able, resourceful, creative and whole, and sets the context for the coaching conversation by valuing the client as central in a very dignified way. In adopting a compassionate approach, the care worker is also affirming that a key motivation of their work is to act at all times to help alleviate the client's suffering. Gilbert and Choden (2014) state that the first attribute of compassion is the deep desire for ourselves and all living things to be free from the cause of suffering. A primary question therefore for the healthcare worker and coach is: how can this coaching conversation serve the client by alleviating suffering?

Step 2 – Allow the client to share their goal and desired outcome

The second step of the coaching process is to help the client clarify their desired goal and to identify a positive outcome from the conversation – essentially, where the client would like to get to at the end of the conversation. By naming this goal, the client reconnects with their needs and the change they wish to make. In seeking simply to understand the client's needs more fully, the care worker coach can help the client to become clearer about what it is that they ideally wish to happen. It may be useful for the care worker to see the setting of the desired goal and positive outcome as a way of developing 'a wellness vision' for the client. This exploration of needs, goals and outcomes commonly offers insight into the client's values, purpose and beliefs. The motivation to change lies in the client being able to express their desired goals in line with their values and to translate these desires, needs and wishes into concrete outcomes. In exploring these values, the care worker may hear the importance of physical, psychological, emotional, environmental, spiritual and social aspects of the client's life.

If we choose to make a fuller assessment of the client's potential resourcefulness in line with their needs, it can be useful to employ motivational interviewing as an effective tool and questionnaire. Cummings *et al.* (2009) show how motivational interviewing focuses on the present, and involves working with a client to access their motivation, with the intention of changing any behaviour that is not consistent with their personal value or goal. To strengthen the client's desired goal, the care worker invites the client to be clear about the outcome they ideally want from the coaching conversation. The work of Hohman and Rollnick (2011), Lundahl and Burke (2009) and Rollnick and Miller

(2002) all support the idea that knowledge alone does not promote change. The key factor is that the client is clear about their motive to change, as well as their knowledge base. When the client is able to describe their desired outcome, they have intentionally placed a solution and end point in mind. The vital coordinates of the coaching compass are then set.

Step 3 – Reflect on current situation and possibilities

Once the client has named their goal, the care worker can, through careful questioning, invite the client to say where they are now and then explore the various possible ways to achieve their desired outcome. What results is an expansion of awareness, as the client seeks to discover, through supported reflection, new potential ways forward to realising their goal. The non-judgemental approach of the care worker respects the fact that the client alone possesses the answer and desired way forward. This permits the simple drawing-out of possible options from the client. During this exploration, the client may find obstacles to achieving their goal. When such limitations arise, it is important to allow the client to name and acknowledge them. The care worker coach can then ask what resources the client may have to overcome such obstacles and move forward.

Step 4 – Empower and enable the client to take action

Having considered the various options, the final stage of the coaching conversation is to empower the client to focus on the specific actions they wish to take as the next practical step or steps. Key questions include:

- What will you do?
- When will you do it by?
- Where will you do it?
- With whom will you do it?

The client names the specific actions that they are willing to take. Note, whereas Step 2 is an expansion, Step 3 is a contraction of awareness – a focusing down on details. It is in this final step that the client's thoughts inform their actions, and move the individual forward towards actually reaching their desired outcome.

Step 1 usually takes the longest, and it is important to get clarity in order to help the client set clear compass bearings for the coaching conversation. In the course of coaching conversations, we may identify a further important need and desire. In this case, we can repeat the process once again – clarifying the key need, drawing out options and agreeing practical steps forward. Rather than seeing these three steps as linear, they may be better represented in the mind's eye in a circular format.

Coaching case study 1: Rita

Begin by reminding yourself of the four-step coaching process and note each step in the following case study:

Step 1 – **C**ompassionate orientation
Step 2 – **A**llow the client to share their goal and desired outcome
Step 3 – **R**eflect upon current situation and possibilities
Step 4 – **E**mpower and enable the client to act.

Rita is an 83-year-old retired schoolteacher. She lives alone in an ordinary terrace house in a small village, where she has lived all her life. When she was 45 years old she was diagnosed with rheumatoid arthritis (a condition that had affected her mother, whom she had nursed towards the end of her life). Over the years, Rita has paid for her own modifications to her home, including a rail from the main road, up seven steps to her front door, and a banister up the staircase leading to her bedroom and bathroom. Downstairs she has installed a gas fire and double-glazing.

Rita has kept in close contact with her GP and in recent months she has been seen by a health visitor, who has suggested that, in view of Rita's age and arthritis, the ground floor be adapted to accommodate her bed as well as a commode. Rita has managed well with appropriate medication over the years.

Following a seven-day stay in hospital, due to complications of bronchitis and suspected pneumonia, a referral has been made for a home assessment. The general feeling amongst the multi-disciplinary team is that Rita needs equipment and some home adaptations to allow her to live as independently as possible.

An occupational therapist (OT) accompanies Rita on a home visit to risk-assess any environmental hazards and see how they can be managed. The OT also plans to identify any equipment required, with a view to encouraging Rita to adapt her home further, enabling her to live downstairs only.

The OT's interview with Rita follows:

The OT is initially thinking about the clinical diagnosis, team concerns and the practical aspects of what might happen and so approaches the conversation from a solely problem-solving perspective.

OT: So Rita, what seems to be the problem here?
Rita: I'm worried that I won't be able to open my front door on my own.
OT: Yes but I hear that you are having problems going upstairs to the toilet. I believe that the health visitor has been to see you and wants you to bring your bed downstairs and have a commode in the living room because of the problem of the stairs.
Rita: I want to sleep upstairs and I don't want a commode in my living room. This is my living room and not my bedroom. I want to carry on going upstairs.
OT: Yes but we all feel that it's getting too difficult for you to go upstairs to your bathroom and bedroom and we'd like to bring things downstairs. Can you show me how you get upstairs?'
Rita manages to get upstairs slowly by holding the banister and then comes downstairs slowly on her backside.

Rita: See this is how I've been getting up and downstairs for a long time.

OT: Yes, I can see that and you have done very well, but why not live downstairs to make things easier and safer for you? Things will get worse and more problems may come up.

Rita: I have been living here all my life and what's important to me is living a normal life, going upstairs to the bathroom and living downstairs in my own way.

Note that the OT's approach is purely problem-directed at this stage. The focus is on the client's condition and diagnosis and the answer put forward by the multi-disciplinary team. At this point, the OT recalls the coaching steps – CARE – and the associated process of caring. Rather than using only a problem-focused approach, she adopts a more compassionate approach. Now the OT starts to consider what might be motivating the client's resistance and decides to employ the four steps.

First, the OT adopts Step 1 – Compassionate approach. Then she moves on to Step 2 – Allow the client to identify the goal and outcome.

OT: So tell me what is working well for you at the moment, Rita.

Rita: I am back in my home, living the way I want to live, having my home as it is, sleeping upstairs and living downstairs.

OT: I can see how important this way of life is to you.

Rita: Yes, it is.

OT: So what is most important to you right now, Rita?

Rita: The minute I lose the capacity to put my own key in the front door, open and lock it behind me, is the day I will choose to die.

OT: I see how very important putting the key in the door is to you.

Rita: Yes, it is. What you have to understand is that I have been going up and down the stairs with my pain for the last 40 years or so and I have adapted to it, and found ways I can make that happen and, although it's more difficult now, I am still able to do it. Doing it each day gives me something to aim for.

OT: So what would you most like out of today?

Rita: Is there anything to help me to put my key in the front door because the arthritis is affecting my hands more and I can't grip the key between my finger and thumb as easy as I could.

Note how the key goal is emerging from the conversation. The OT now moves to the next step and starts to consider Step 3 – Reflect on the current situation and possibilities.

OT: Let's explore options and what we might do together to help. Have you any ideas about how you might move this forward?

Rita: I have tried holding the key in different ways but I can't hold it well now and it often slips – I am frightened that one day soon I might not be able to open the door.

OT: I understand your feelings. So you have tried holding it in different ways?

Rita: Yes I have.

OT: Anything else?

Rita: I've been wondering if I might be able to put the key in something so I can hold it better?

OT: That's a good idea. If we found something to help with this, what difference would it make to you, Rita?

Rita: It would give me back my independence and a belief that I can still live in my own home.

OT: Let's see what we can do to help make this happen. I have an idea that we might be able to put the key into something that you can hold better and, from listening to you, I think this would really help.

The OT examines Rita holding a small orange. Placing the key in the small orange, the OT observes that Rita is able to grip better and insert and turn the key in her front door more successfully. The OT explains that she will return with an adapted wooden ball, with the key securely fixed in it, which will allow Rita to grip the key more easily and unlock her front door.

OT: I will come back shortly with this for you and we can make sure it works.

Rita: You have no idea what that would mean to me... It's a godsend and I feel so much better, having spoken to you about it.

Finally, the OT moves on to Step 4 – Empower and enable the client to act.

OT: So what's the next step, Rita?

Rita: Thank you for your help in giving me something to allow me to grip better and open the door. I will feel more independent and I will use it every day without fail.

OT: We seem to have found what's important to you and helped you to move forward.

Rita: You have, you truly have... Thank you.

A home assessment was made and Rita was found to be safe and able to live alone and independently.

Coaching case study 2: Martin

Peter is a nurse working in palliative care. Martin is a new patient. He has recently been diagnosed with cancer and is uncertain of the extent of his diagnosis. Peter notices that Martin is looking down and a little depressed. Peter is attending to his basic hygiene care and adopts a compassionate orientation (Step 1).

Nurse: Martin, I have noticed that you seem a little down? How are you feeling?

Martin: Yes, I am a little down. I find myself regretting things.

Nurse: May I ask what you are regretting?

Martin: Missed opportunities in life.

Nurse: Missed opportunities?

Martin: Yes, there are things I would have loved to have done, and I am not sure I will get to do them now.

Nurse: Would doing these things help you at this time?

Martin: I believe so. I want to be happier at this challenging time and not down, although I know sometimes I will be down.

Nurse: I am interested in what you are saying. Are you willing to talk a little more?

Martin: Yes – I would like to say more.

Nurse: And from our conversation today, what would you like to walk away with?

Notice that Peter has recognised the goal that Martin wants to work on – Martin regrets having missed out on things in life and wants to make some sort of change. Peter now invites Martin to identify an ideal outcome from their conversation (Step 2).

Martin: Mmm (pauses), one or two important things that would help me through this period.

Nurse: So, one or two things, yeah? How will we know when you get there?

Martin: Laughs. I will feel happier, more in control and as if I am moving forward.

Nurse: What would that feel like?

Martin: Much better.

Notice how clear Martin becomes about his desired outcome through Peter's questioning, to the extent that he knows how he will feel and what that will give him.

Nurse: Sounds like a good place for you to get to. So tell me, where would you like to begin?

Martin: I want to acknowledge the things that are important to me now.

Nurse: Go for it.

Martin: My loved ones are essential to me – my partner Julie, most especially. I want to plan something special for us to do together. Not big, but quality. I know she will be very worried but I want to be able to tell her how much I value her and about the great times we have had so far and hopefully ones to come.

Nurse: Sounds important, any ideas?

Now Peter is exploring options with Martin (Step 3).

Martin: I want to take her for a meal each month, somewhere special. Just for us to put everything else down and to have a good time – and enjoy ourselves, despite my illness. I will get through it if I stay positive.

Nurse: So you'd like a monthly meal with your partner and the chance for quality time and for you to be positive.

Martin: Yes, that's it. Also, I want to be able to plan something I have never done before, for when I am through this.

Nurse: Sounds important and interesting.

Martin: I want to take a trip back to one of my favourite places on earth – the Maldives – with Julie. When we first met we went there, and I would love to go back. Money and other things have put me off but it will be the perfect place to be together and for me to recuperate properly.

Nurse: What will the Maldives trip give you?

Martin: A chance to plan for a better time and to do something that will take away my regrets about potentially missed opportunities, a chance to really heal in a place that is special to both of us.

Nurse: When will your trip be?

At this point, Peter is enabling Martin to become clear about his actions (Step 4).

Martin: I can't decide for sure because it depends on my surgery and treatment but, as soon as I am aware of my schedule, I will start planning and I will start putting money aside and looking forward to the prospect.

Nurse: What will this planning give you?

Martin: Something to truly look forward to and to get me through this period of uncertainty.

Nurse: How are you feeling now, with these plans?

Martin: So much better, so much better.

Nurse: How come? Smiling.

Martin: I feel I've taken charge at a challenging time and I am now saying 'yes' to life. I am going to help myself through this and value what I have now and plan something important for the future. I know I will feel down sometimes but these plans will help me.

Nurse: You said you wanted to walk away feeling happier, more in control and moving forward – how are you doing?

Notice that Peter is checking with Martin about whether he feels he is reaching his desired outcome.

Martin: Good, very good – I feel happier and that I do have some control and I am moving forward.

Nurse: So, what are your next steps?

For clarity, Peter now repeats and affirms Step 4 – empowering and enabling the client to act.

Martin: I am going to share all my plans with Julie today. I have a restaurant in mind for this month.

Nurse: Great. Well done, Martin! Can I check in on you from time to time and see how your plans are going?

Martin: That would be great. Thanks for this conversation and your time. I really appreciate it.

The key qualities and skills of the care worker coach

In this section we explore the key skills and qualities that emerge when the care worker becomes a more appreciative practitioner. These qualities inform and support their coaching activity.

Being present

The degree to which the care worker is able to give their attention to the client is a measure of the extent to which their presence is felt. As their presence builds, the care worker is experienced as being more available, attentive and in service of the client. The care worker's presence is expressed in their non-judgemental, accepting attitude. Gilbert and Choden (2014, p. 217) note that the 'primary objective of acceptance is our moment-by-moment experience rather than what caused the experience behind it'. This contrasts with the experiential avoidance that is characteristic of the unawakened analytical eye. Chawla and Ostafin (2007, p. 871) describe this as an 'unwillingness to remain in contact with private experiences such as painful thoughts and emotions'. Knowing that the care worker is attentive and available naturally builds rapport, engagement and trust in the relationship. Being no longer largely distracted, the care worker demonstrates poise and ease, and a sense that they are calm and collected.

As we have seen, the presence of the care worker can be developed through mindfulness practice (as detailed in Chapter 7). The practitioner's capacity to inwardly reflect and bear witness, developing sensitivity to their thoughts and feelings, also enables them to accommodate the thoughts and feelings of the client. Presence allows the care worker to remain attentive to the client through the coaching conversation, and develops sympathy and empathy. In this context, sympathy refers to a heightened sense of another's need and potential suffering, and empathy is an ability to focus awareness on another's experience in order to understand them better (Gilbert & Choden 2014, p. 110). Throughout the coaching conversation, the care worker is not imposing their viewpoint or making critical judgements but drawing out the client's own experience and solutions. Once more, the analogy of driving a car is useful. During the coaching conversation, the care worker is sitting in the passenger seat, whilst the client is always in the driving seat, setting their own goals and discovering their own best option to move forward with the actions that they choose to implement.

Seeing potential and possibility

Whenever we are working with a client as an appreciative care worker and coach, we are invited to look beyond where the client is currently, to see future possibility and potential. As we saw earlier, in Step 1 of the coaching conversation, the care worker coach approaches the client with a belief in their wholeness, creativity and innate resourcefulness. This enables the care worker to develop with the client a vision of potential wellness, giving the client the opportunity to recall and align with their more resourceful self. Potentiality, and the client's motivation to change, is realised in helping the client to create this vision.

A curiosity to question and a wish to understand

With the ending of impulsiveness, qualities can quite naturally emerge that inform the work of the carer. When we are not compelled to get to the answer, we discover instead a growing curiosity and deeper interest in both self and others that motivates inquiry. These are essential relational qualities that inform the care worker's intention to get to know and understand the client's needs better and to offer care that is aimed at relieving suffering. This builds the ability to listen and question.

The unawakened analytical eye, as you will recall, is compelled to answer and will commonly tell the client what to do. In contrast, the appreciative care worker recognises the client's value and potential resourcefulness and asks questions rather than giving instructions. Dembkowski *et al.* (2006) note that good questions usually have three features. They are:

- Simple
- Asked with a specific purpose in mind
- Designed to have a positive impact.

Generally, the care worker coach employs open and/or probing questions. A key purpose of the coaching conversation is to expand the client's awareness while helping them discover new options and ultimately informing new choices. This necessitates the use of open and probing questions.

Open questions are those that we do not answer with a simple 'yes' or 'no', such as:

- What would be useful?
- What are your needs at the moment?
- What are your options?
- What resources do you have?

Probing questions are often short and simple, and invite the client to explore the topic in question more deeply or broadly. They may include:

- Can you say any more?
- Anything else?
- What more will you do?

Closed questions are used only rarely in the coaching conversation and usually relate specifically to goal setting or practical action planning:

- Is this the goal you want to explore?
- Are you able to do this?

Questions starting with 'why' are only rarely used, since they are often experienced by the client as judgemental. This type of question tends to push the client into re-evaluation, rather than expanding their awareness and options.

The action planning part of the coaching conversation is very practical and 'what', 'when' and 'where' are very useful questions for the care worker coach to ask at this stage. For example:

- What will you do next?
- When will you do it?
- Where is this going to happen?

The capacity to listen with empathy

As the care worker develops presence, they become more able to tune into the client's subjective experience. With this capacity to develop empathy comes the opportunity to practise listening. Note that listening (as opposed to hearing) is an applied and active skill. When the care worker listens, they are processing and making sense of what they are hearing. Note how our capacity to listen changes markedly when we view our caring practice through the three lenses of our three-eye model:

- Analytical eye – distracted or partial listening
- Appreciative eye – listening for understanding
- Creative eye – listening for potential and possibility.

The analytical eye offers only a very limited form of distracted listening. Recall how, in employing this lens, the care worker is commonly preoccupied with the voice of their inner critic and judge. This distracts attention away from the client and onto the care worker. Clues to the distracted listening of the practitioner include evidence of reactivity and attempts to multi-task, lack of eye contact and the compulsion to answer rather than question. With the opening of the appreciative eye, the capacity to listen develops, as the care worker becomes more reflective and empathic. The practitioner is now able to check for understanding by clarifying assumptions, and mirroring or repeating back the client's key words or phrases. The appreciative healthcare worker is thus able to listen and check for understanding. With the opening of the creative eye, the true art and practice of listening in the care worker coach reaches its fullest development and application.

Rogerian theory (Heppener, Rogers & Lee 1984) recognises that, for the client to learn and grow, it is important for the practitioner to be able to listen with acceptance and without judgement. With non-judgemental acceptance, the care worker coach learns how to listen more deeply, and to consider the client's story behind their words and what may remain unspoken. This 'listening for hidden potential' often reveals what is most important to the client, expressing their true values, beliefs and sense of purpose. In sharing this awareness, the client gets the opportunity to recall and/or discover key strengths, values and more positive and empowering beliefs that combine to inform and motivate the positive change they wish to make.

Being an authentic mirror

Peltier (2010, p. 104) examines the three vital characteristics that promote the client's growth, in accordance with the work of Rogers:

- Congruence and genuineness
- Unconditional positive regard and acceptance
- An accurate empathic understanding.

Peltier (2010, p. 105) also guides the practitioner to try 'to walk in the shoes of the client by reflecting, with sensitivity and accuracy'. This reminds us that a key aspect of the work of the appreciative practitioner is to develop the capacity to be an authentic mirror. As well as repeating the client's key words and phrases to check engagement and understanding, the care worker coach will also at times mirror back what they sense and intuit in order to help the client to realise their own hidden potential. In being authentic, the care worker creates a relationship where both parties treat each other with respect and tell the truth as it is experienced. Block (2000, p. 37) describes how 'authentic behaviour with a client means you put into words what you are experiencing with the client as you work. This is the most powerful thing that you can do to leverage what you are looking for and to build client commitment'.

Being compassionate – acting to relieve suffering

In Chapters 1, 6 and 7 we explored the relationship between empathy and compassion in healthcare practice. Kanov *et al.* (2004) note there are three elements to compassion in practice:

- Developing the interrelationship of practitioner and client and an attention to and a noticing of suffering in the present moment
- An empathic concern involving a 'suffering with' the client
- A willingness to respond to lessening, alleviating or making suffering more bearable.

It is important to recall here that compassion adds an active or directional element to the empathic approach of the care worker, reminding us that the intention is always to act in order to relieve or lessen suffering. Through the creative eye's capacity to offer responsive person-centred care, the care worker can combine empathy from the appreciative eye with the practical and planning skills of the awakened analytical eye, and model all three elements of compassionate practice. Fogarty *et al.* (1999) showed that a compassionate approach to healthcare reduced patient anxiety, and Taylor (1997) illustrated how compassion fostered positive patient outcomes. Compassion also appears to bring about a positive upward spiral. Goetz *et al.* (2010) report that clients receiving compassion are subsequently better able or more likely to demonstrate caring and supportive behaviour towards others.

Being dignified

Adler (1993) reminds us of a central premise that any human being has an innate right to be valued and to receive ethical treatment. Practitioners working with dignity avoid harm and always offer assistance to foster the client's well-being. The care worker is invited to remember at all times the worth of the client. The word dignity derives from the Latin *dignitas*, meaning 'worthiness'. Its modern use often suggests that someone is not receiving the proper degree of respect or may even be lacking in self-respect. As the care worker develops their self-respect as a practitioner, they become equally aware of the need to value and respect others. A key aspect of the role of the appreciative practitioner, and step 1 of our coaching process, is to affirm the value of the client. Sincere statements of affirmation and belief in the client enable them to recall their own value and worth, despite whatever challenging circumstances they may be facing. Such affirmations support the client in moving forward with their intention to realise their desired goals and be more resourceful.

The vital role of supervision for the care worker and coach

Gilbert and Choden (2014, p. 300) remind us that 'without training the powerful drives of the pleasure seeking resource demanding drive system and the anxious and aggressive threat system [in our model, approaching caring through the unawakened analytical eye] can run the show'. Furthermore (p. 301), they state that 'the compassionate self requires our attention, training and cultivation'. A key question is: what resources does the care worker coach have to support them in this vital task?

We believe that individual and group supervision can be an essential resource to support the development of the compassionate and responsive care worker. Regular clinical supervision meetings are commonly employed in many disciplines within the healthcare system. Supervision is a vital forum where the care worker can discuss their casework and other professional challenges in a structured and supported way with an experienced supervisor.

Supervision will often emphasise the client's clinical diagnosis and focus on exploring the practitioner's technical and specialist expertise. However, it can equally well be used as an opportunity to explore the continuing development of the care worker's coaching skills and qualities. Within a context of extended scope practice, supervision is a safe and supportive environment where key limitations and challenges faced by the care worker can be disclosed to reveal what may have been hidden.

According to Cochrane and Newton (2011, p. 2), supervision is: 'a place of possibility and safety, without personal judgement, where learning is noticed and recognised and competence brought into awareness: a place where both partners (supervisor and care worker) can be truthful, where there is a joy in learning and no shame in disclosure; a collegial relationship where there is authenticity, a balance of power and both parties are absolutely accepted'.

This reminds us that a key goal of supervision is to develop well-informed and well-trained care workers who are intent on, and supported in, developing personal coaching skills and qualities. Supervision should also help care workers explore any ethical issues that arise in their work, as well as fostering technical excellence and expertise. The relationship between the care worker and client can be explored developmentally, alongside consideration of the wider organisational culture. Kadushin and Harknes (2002) identify three key values of supervision:

- To support
- To develop
- To manage.

Cochrane and Newton (2011) recognise that the supportive aspect of supervision should allow the practitioner to identify their own learning needs and any risks of collusion, burn-out and somatic reactions to stress. Equally, the supervision session should identify what is working well, and affirm the practitioner in their willingness to learn and develop. Supervision can be conducted either one-to-one or within a group setting. The advantage of the group is that it offers an amplified opportunity for support, learning and shared development. The care worker develops according to their willingness to work with and reveal both their limitations and their strengths. The management aspect of supervision reminds us of the importance of being able to bring forth and discuss any ethical considerations, and the need to examine and validate coaching work and identify key steps to continually improve coaching practice.

Conclusion

This chapter has highlighted the key emergent skills and qualities that naturally lead to coaching conversations, which are vital to the daily practice of compassionate person-centred care. We presented a four-step coaching process that can be employed by any care worker. This CARE process was developed and explained in detail. Its key steps are: adopting a Compassionate orientation, Allowing the client to name their desired goal and outcome, Reflecting on the current situation and future possibilities; and Empowering the client to act and move forward.

We also illustrated how such coaching conversations fully engage and empower the client to self-manage and self-care, whilst developing their resourcefulness, accountability and confidence. Supervision is recognised as a vital resource to validate, support and develop the care worker's personal skills and coaching approach, whilst also accommodating the technical and professional aspects of their role. In this way, we can achieve a continual expansion of the care worker's awareness – a 'SUPER-VISION' – that sustains the work of the appreciative healthcare worker as a compassionate, person-centred coach and carer.

Chapter 9

Conclusion

'To care for someone, I must know many things. I must know, for example, who the other is, what his powers and limitations are, what his needs are, and what is conducive to his growth; I must know how to respond to his needs, and what my own powers and limitations are.'
(Mayeroff 1971 p. 19)

This book has raised many questions. Our purpose was not to form a theory, system or unifying philosophy of experience and consciousness. Rather, we sought to describe a very specific human ability – how to become aware of the client's needs and desires, and thereby come to know and to care. Some may rationalise a care worker's absence of concern, compassion and dignity by saying that they are 'being a good professional' by not getting too involved with individual clients. Such an attitude may be partly understandable as a stress management approach, but it is not an acceptable or satisfactory response to the most basic human need – to be cared for. It also flies in the face of the many healthcare strategies and policies that highlight the importance of both compassion and care.

Having said this, when the media constantly criticise the NHS, it tends to increase fear and anxiety amongst care workers. Our reaction to this continual criticism can often contribute to our lack of caring. As a result, society's reaction to extreme examples of lack of care is likely to compound the problem, rather than relieve it. Of course lack of care should be revealed whenever it occurs. But when was the last time we read about success in the NHS and how often do we hear about best practice and excellence in care? Do we only see the problems and remain blind to the successes? This book argues for the vital importance of opening a more appreciative eye and viewpoint on the whole system as well as our individual practice within it.

When we apply a less limited and more responsive approach to finding solutions, we give the client the opportunity to take responsibility for framing their own problem, and thus engage and learn for themselves. This 'self-learning' forms a new, key aspect of problem resolution and person-centred practice, and we thereby become relational facilitators and solution-focused problem-solvers – in other words, a care coach. By shifting our role from instructor or technical expert to coach, we can continually develop and inform higher-level practice. In practising an appreciative and creative approach, our practice becomes truly person-centred, while at the same time inviting the application of technical and clinical expertise. Our hope is that practitioners will start cultivating both personal and professional competencies and, through continual development and supervision, learn how to balance them equally. Growing numbers of appreciative, creative and person-centred care workers will in turn influence the whole culture of health and social care.

Rising to the challenge

One key question that has emerged in writing this book is how we can learn to offer a thoughtful, compassionate and dignified response to the challenges we face as professional carers. Sadly, there is evidence of uncaring practice and even extreme patient abuse and unnecessary death within the care system. This realisation may instil a sense of horror in everyone. But it would be a mistake to reactively locate the problem (and blame) in a few individual care workers, who are found to be unprofessional and assumed to be very different from the rest of us. In this book, we have illustrated the importance of bringing the issue of compassion home, as the central responsibility of every care worker. We have shown, through the application of the three-eye model, how we can all become uncaring in our practice. It may be tempting to deny or dismiss this fact, but acknowledging its validity is vital to the continued development of care work and sustaining best practice. Rather than being trapped (as we so often are) in the partial vision of the analytical eye, judging practice as simply 'good' or 'bad', we need to start seeing a continuum of care, ranging from reactive and uncaring to responsive, compassionate, person-centred care.

Only by accepting personal accountability for our own care practice, and being willing to own our vulnerabilities as well as our strengths as care workers, will we be able to acknowledge the vital resources that we need to care with compassion and to develop a more compassionate culture in healthcare. Denying personal accountability and so locating the problem outside, rather than within, only compounds the pressure that can potentially lead to inadequate care. In order to be attentive to others and to care responsively, to see our clients as whole beings beyond their diagnosis, to be motivated to meet their needs with an intent to relieve suffering, we must first learn how to respect and care for ourselves as practitioners.

Conclusion

Self-caring, not selfishness

A core principle of this approach is that caring starts with the practitioner and then naturally extends to the client. One cannot proceed without the other, and the two types of caring are mutually interdependent. We must not confuse this central principle with being selfishly concerned about ourselves. This type of self-caring is quite the opposite of selfishness; understanding the practice and meaning of self-care is in fact a necessity for all carers. Without this understanding, we can end up compulsively (through the limited and emotionally driven vision of the unawakened analytical eye) over-caring for others as an over-compensating reaction to the lack of care for ourselves. In doing so, we create an unhealthy approach and a profoundly unbalanced healthcare system.

To develop best practice in care, we need to learn to speak truthfully about our experience (including our limitations and fears, against the background of our strengths) and feel supported to look within ourselves to discover the necessary resourcefulness to respond, rather than react. Coaching and supervisory relationships can, when properly developed, help care workers sustain person-centred, compassionate care. The problem is very rarely bad practitioners (though this may appear to be the case); it is more often we as practitioners who are unable to own, and lack the courage to speak out, about what is limiting our practice.

Current fear of litigation may compound the issue, and increased regulation can silence the carer's voice. Once more, supervision (with a balance of personal and professional considerations) is a vital resource. These sessions enable the carer to build up enough trust to speak out about work pressures and their sense of their own limitations. They can also be supported in facing any fears, guilt and shame. Only by working with these emotions do we recall the deeper values and beliefs that inform our sense of purpose and the very reason why we choose to care. Alternatively, if we react to pressure of work and see our clients as potential threats, we can easily hide in the shadow of the analytical eye, carrying out reactive, uncaring practice.

Moving forward

To care compassionately, we have to care enough to take an appreciative step out into the open and own our own limitations, whilst equally acknowledging the supportive, motivational platform of our strengths. In moving forward, should we judge the caring chain by its weakest or its strongest link? When combined, both are equally vital. As we have seen, being able to consciously open a creative eye and step into being a compassionate practitioner brings several essential qualities and capabilities to our practice, including:

- An ability to be fully attentive towards another, fostering rapport, trust, engagement and relationship

- A capacity to listen deeply and question (rather than tell), due to an expanded bandwidth of awareness
- An ability to gain a clearer, fuller picture of current reality and client needs, desires and aspirations
- An ability to see the client as a whole creative person, beyond their clinical diagnosis
- An interest in seeking to understand our clients as human beings like ourselves
- A growing awareness of our clients' potential and how this can be realised through care as a vital aspect of healing
- A capacity to enable and empower the client to self-care, develop and become more resourceful, despite their diagnosis and illness
- An ability to step into a more compassionate approach to care as the first step in all coaching conversations, while being motivated to relieve suffering and maintain the dignity of the individual
- A capacity to develop a social conscience as a care worker that fosters more collaborative working and an integrated response to client need and care
- An opportunity to learn how to care for ourselves, as a measure of the extent to which we can care for others.

In transforming need to desired outcome, the creative eye of the care worker can enliven and harness the hidden potential and resourcefulness of both the practitioner and the client. Many of our care colleagues speak outside their work of what can't be spoken within, such as the setting of unrealistic targets by managers and leaders who appear to have somehow become detached from the coalface of caring. The resulting care strategies are the antithesis of compassion – driven purely by over-ambitious efficiency and cost-cutting targets. Without keeping the word 'compassion' as our touchstone in everyday practice and the wider healthcare system, we can end up unconsciously defaulting (through the unawakened analytical eye) to uncaring practice and its inhumane consequences. Let compassion replace competition.

Transforming limitations into strengths

In conclusion, a central thesis that has emerged through this book is that our limitations, if owned and accepted, can change to become our greatest strengths – our lock is in fact a vital key. If we can remember and speak of our strengths first, we then have a platform to build upon and to support our limitations. And in doing so, we will find the missing resource we need to care. Only by witnessing and attending to our own needs, and resisting the compulsion to problem-solve, can we rediscover our motivation and resourcefulness to care, and mark an end in ourselves to the prospect of uncaring practice. In a healthcare system that strategically seeks to offer compassion and dignity to our clients, we are first invited to show the same compassion and dignity to ourselves as care workers. Once more, only in learning how to respond (and resist the temptation to react) can we model compassion and dignity in practice. In doing so, we will reap the rewards of clients feeling more empowered and resourceful and even becoming able to take their own personal steps to return to well-being.

The true nature of caring

Caring is the very antithesis of telling or instructing. The approach of management in setting vital targets, managing performance and results, the sharing of important experiences through mentoring relationships, all have their place within the healthcare system. However, empowering our clients through coaching conversations is the only way to draw out hidden potential and resourcefulness that is vital to the care system as a whole. In addition, we have to learn how to show empathy whilst retaining an element of detached care in order to help realise the client's goal and relieve suffering. It is important to look at this in a little more detail. How do we actually define caring in practice?

A number of practitioners have spoken to us about what they call 'caring burn-out' and the danger of what they perceive to be 'over-caring'. The analytical eye can often judge those who are ill as somehow inferior: 'how sad/what a pity/poor them'. When we consider an illness such as cancer, for example, an immediate reaction may be to offer pity and sympathy. A sympathetic act may appear caring on the surface, but is it in fact wholly in service of the client? What truly serves the client is seeing beyond what they present, and perceiving them as healthy and whole in our mind's eye. In this way, we can help them to access their own resourcefulness and resilience. Whilst acknowledging the impact of potential trauma and illness and listening intently, we should ask questions like:

- What will sustain you through this period?
- What is most important to you now?
- What resources do you have?
- How will you be engaged in your care?

All these questions encourage the client towards a more empowered and engaged position.

At the heart of caring is an empathic, compassionate, rather than over-sympathetic, attitude. If we only sympathise, we can end up disempowering the client by trying to be over-helpful rather than useful. Working with compassion, you will recall the importance of what we called 'objective intimacy', an attitude of focused attention, presence and non-judgemental acceptance that seeks to end suffering wherever possible by enabling the client to rediscover their own resourcefulness and vitality. This attitude allows us to share in the client's experience, whilst always maintaining a slight distance that allows us to facilitate the recognition and implementation of the client's desired choices.

To genuinely care, we need to be responsive to (and implicitly in service of) the client. And to be so, we have to recognise how at times we might unintentionally collude and disempower. As carers, we are invited to respond to the client and not react; or to become aware of reaction and instead choose to respond. This detachment as an aspect of enabling caring is truly compassionate and in marked contrast to 'killing someone with kindness'. In a misguided need to merge with, and inadvertently devalue a client, we can end up smothering them and depriving them of a vital opportunity to contribute to their own healing.

All this has led us to define caring as a compassionate and dignified responsiveness in practice that is ever in service of the client becoming more resourceful, whole, healthy and self-caring. Clinically, we require that things be done to us as patients – expert procedures, therapy, interventions, the prescribing of medication. But as practitioners, we must be able to see the innate potential and resourcefulness of the client. Through the creative eye, we can develop this intimate objectivity, this ability to detach with care in order to show compassion. In this book, we offer all practitioners a guide to how we can become more person-centred, compassionate and dignified carers. In applying our model, we hope you will gain the necessary insight, awareness and learning and realise that you can continue to develop a more mindful, person-centred caring practice, despite the pressures of work. The development of the care coach is a vital personal (as well as team and organisational) resource. What would the impact be if all healthcare systems were to support and enable the development of coaching skills in all carers? Furthermore, can we develop a cadre of vocational care coaches as an essential internal conscience and resource to sustain compassionate care?

A final question that has emerged from writing this book is: do we all have the capacity to be care workers? Is caring actually the vocation of some but not all? We believe this is a vital decision that each individual must make – in the clear-eyed knowledge of all their own limitations, vulnerabilities and strengths. The best we can do is to be fully aware of the responsibility and opportunity of caring. If our role is a caring one, we can never excuse a lack of compassion and care. We invite you to make this choice for yourself.

References

Adler, M.J. (1993). *The Difference of Man and the Difference It Makes*. The Bronx, New York: Fordham University Press.

Allen, K.D. & Hancock, T.E. (2008). Reading comprehension improvement with individualised cognitive profiles and metacognition. *Literacy Research and Instruction*. **47** (2), 124–39.

Andrews Report (2014). Trusted to Care: An Independent Review of the Princess of Wales Hospital and Neath Port Talbot Hospital at Abertawe Bro Morgannwg University Health Board. http://wales.gov.uk/docs/dhss/publications/140512trustedtocareen.pdf (Accessed 12 June 2014).

Baker, R. (2013). A Review of Deaths of Patients at Gosport War Memorial Hospital. https://www.gov.uk/government/uploads/system/uploads/attachment_data/file/226263/review_gosport_war_memorial_hospital.pdf (Accessed 14 October 2013).

Ball, J., Murrells, T., Rafferty, A.M., Morrow, E. & Griffiths, P. (2013). 'Care left undone' during nursing shifts: associations with workload and perceived quality of care. *British Medical Journal for Quality and Safety*. doi:10.1136/bmjqs-2012-001767

Barrows, H.S. (2000). *Problem-Based Learning Applied to Medical Education*. Springfield, Illinois: Southern Illinois University School of Medicine.

Baumeister, R.F. (1991). *Meanings of Life*. New York City: Guilford Press.

Baumeister, R.F., Bratslavsky, E., Finkenauer, C. & Vohs, K.D. (2001). Bad is stronger than good. *Review of General Psychology*. **5** (4), 323–70.

Baumeister, R.F., Bratslavsky, E., Muraven, M. & Tice, D. (1998). Ego depletion – is the active self a limited resource? *Journal of Personality and Social Psychology*. **75** (5), 1252–65.

Bechtel, C. & Ness, D.L. (2010). If you build it, will they come? Designing truly patient-centered healthcare. *Health Affairs*. **29** (5), 914–20.

Berwick, D., Bibby, J., Bisognano, M., Callaghan, I., Dalton, D., Dixon-Woods, M., Gould, J., Haraden, C., Hartley, J., Ingelsby-Burke, E., Leaper, L., Leggot, J., Leitch, J., Reason, J.T., Singleton, S. & Vincent, C. (2013). *A promise to learn – a commitment to act. Improving the safety of patients in England*. London: National Advisory group on safety of patients in England.

Biggs, J.B. (2003). *Teaching for Quality Learning at University*. (2nd edn). SHRE & Open University Press.

Block, P. (2000). *Flawless Consulting: A guide to getting your expertise used*. (2nd edn). San Francisco, California: Jossey-Bass/Pfeiffer.

Boud, D. & Feletti, G. (eds) (1997). 'Part 1: what is problem-based learning?' in *The Challenge of Problem-Based Learning*. London: Kogan Page, 15–16.

Boyd, N.M. & Bright, D.S. Bright (2007). Appreciative inquiry as a mode of action research for a community psychology. *Journal of Community Psychology*. **35** (8).

Brickman, P. (1987). *Handbook of Motivation and Cognition*. New York City: The Guilford Press.

Cairns, D., Williams, V., Victor, C., Richards, S., Le May, A., Martin, W. & Oliver, D. (2013). The meaning and importance of dignified care: findings from a survey of health and social care professionals. *BMC Geriatrics*. **13** (28).

Calnan, M., Badcott, D. & Woolhead, G. (2006). Dignity under threat? A study of the experiences of older people in the United Kingdom. *The International Journal of Health Service*. **36** (2), 355–75.

Cameron, K.S., Dutton, J.E. & Quinn, R.E. (2003). *Positive Organizational Scholarship – foundations of a new discipline*. San Francisco: Berrett-Kochler Publishers Inc.

Care Quality Commission (2011). *Dignity and Nutrition Inspection Programme. National Overview*. http://www.cqc.org.uk/content/national-report-dignity-and-nutrition-review-published (Accessed 10 May 2015).

Chaskalson, M. (2011). *The Mindful Workplace – Developing Resilient Individuals and Resonant Organisations with MBSR*. Chichester, UK: Wiley and Sons Ltd.

Chawla, N. & Ostafin, B.(2007). Experiential avoidance as a functional dimensional approach to psychopathology: An empirical review. *Journal of Clinical Psychology*. **63** (9), 871–90.

Clarke, M. & Thornton, J. (2014). Using appreciative inquiry to explore the potential of enhanced practice education opportunities. *The British Journal of Occupational Therapy*. **77** (9), 475–78.

Cloke, K. & Goldsmith, J. (2006). *The Art of Waking People up – Cultivating Awareness and Authenticity at Work*. San Franscisco, California: Jossey-Bass.

Cochrane, H. & Newton, T. (2011). *Supervision for Coaches – a guide to thoughtful work*. Ipswich, UK: Supervision for Coaches.

Cooperrider, D. & Srivastva, R. (1987). 'Appreciative Inquiry in Organizational Life' in R. Woodman & W. Pasmore (eds) *Research on Organizational Change and Development*. **1**. Greenwich CT: JAI Press.

Cooperrider, D.L. & Whitney, D. (2000). 'A Positive Revolution in Change: Appreciative Inquiry' in D. Cooperrider, P.F. Sorensen, D. Whitney & T.F. Yaeger (eds) *Appreciative Inquiry: Rethinking Human Organization Toward a Positive Theory of Change*. Champaign, Illinois: Stripes Publishing.

Cooperrider, D.L. & Whitney, D. (2005). *Appreciative Inquiry: a positive revolution in change*. San Francisco, California: Berrett-Koehler Publishers Inc.

Creek, J. (2010). *The Core Concepts of Occupational Therapy: A Dynamic Framework for Practice*. London: Jessica Kingsley Publishers.

Crossley, J., Humphris, G. & Jolly, B. (2002). Accessing health professionals. *Medical Education*. 36, 800–804.

Csikszentmihalyi, M. (1992). *Flow: The psychology of happiness*. London: Rider and Co.

Cummings, S.M., Cooper, R.L. & Cassie, K.M. (2009). Motivational interviewing to affect behavioral change in older adults. *Research on Social Work Practice*. **19** (2), 195–204.

Dane, E. (2011). Paying attention to mindfulness and its effects on task performance in the workplace. *Journal of Management*. **37** (4), 997–1018.

Dembkowski, S., Eldridge, F. & Hunter, I. (2006). *The Seven Steps of Effective Executive Coaching*. London: Thorogood.

Department of Health (2000a). *A strategy for the allied health professions. Meeting the Challenge*. London: The Stationery Office.

Department of Health (2000b). *The NHS Plan: a plan for investment, a plan for reform. Cmnd4880*. London: The Stationery Office.

Department of Health (2001). https://www.gov.uk/government/publications/quality-standards-for-care-services-for-older-people (Accessed 19 April 2015).

References

Department of Health (2011). *The Operating Framework for the NHS in England 2012–13.* https://www.gov.uk/government/publications/the-operating-framework-for-the-nhs-in-england-2012-13 (Accessed 19 April 2015).

Department of Health (2012). *Deprivation of Liberty Safeguards (DOLS) Funding Fact-Sheet for 2013/14.* https://www.gov.uk/government/publications/department-publishes-deprivation-of-liberty-safeguards-funding-factsheet (Accessed 9 June 2013).

Dilts, R. (2003). *From Coach to Awakener.* California, USA: Meta Publications.

Dixon-Woods, M., Baker, R., Charles, K., Dawson, J., Jerzembek, G., Martin, G., McCarthy, I., McKee, L., Minion, J., Ozieranski, P., Willars, J., Wilkie, P. & West, M. (2013). Culture and behaviour in the English National Health Service: overview of lessons from a large multi method study. *British Medical Journal of Quality & Safety.* doi:10.1136/bmjqs-2013-001947

Downey, M. (2003). *Effective Coaching – Lessons from the Coach's Coach.* (2nd edn). Mason, Ohio: Orion Business.

Edmonstone, J. (2006). *Building on the Best – An Introduction to Appreciative Inquiry in Healthcare.* Chichester, Sussex: Kingsham Press.

Evans, R. & Russell, P. (1989). *The Creative Manager.* London: Unwin HarperCollins Publishers Ltd.

Faulkner, A. & Sweeney, A. (2011). *Prevention in Adult Safeguarding: A review of the literature.* London: Social Care Institute for Excellence.

Fitzgerald., S.P., Murrell, K.L. & Newman, H.L. (2001). 'Appreciative inquiry – the new frontier' in J. Waclawski & A.H. Church (eds) *Organization Development: Data driven methods for change.* San Francisco: Jossey-Bass Publishers, 203–21.

Fogarty, L.A., Curbow, B.A., Wingard, J.R., McDonnell, K. & Somerfield, M.R. (1999). Can 40 seconds of compassion reduce patient anxiety? *Journal of Clinical Oncology.* **17**, 371–79.

Francis, R. (2013). *Report of the Mid Staffordshire NHS Foundation Trust Public Inquiry: The Mid Staffordshire NHS Foundation Trust. Public Inquiry.* London: The Stationery Office.

Fredrickson, B.L. (1998). What good are positive emotions? *Review of General Psychology.* **2**, 300–319.

Fredrickson, B.L. (2001). The role of positive emotions in positive psychology. *American Psychologist.* **56** (3), 218–26

Fredrickson, B.L. (2003). 'Chapter 11: Positive Emotions and Upward Spirals in Organizations' in K.S. Cameron, J.E. Dutton & R.E. Quinn (2003). *Positive Organizational Scholarship – Foundations of a New Discipline.* San Francisco: Berrett-Kochler Publishers Inc.

Gaffney, M. (2011). *Flourishing – how to achieve a deeper sense of well-being, meaning and purpose – even when facing adversity.* London: Penguin Books Ltd.

Gallwey, T. (2000). *The Inner Game of Work.* New York: Random House Inc.

Gazzaninga, M.S. (1985). *The Social Brain.* New York: Basic Books.

Gazzaninga, M.S. (1993). 'Brain mechanisms and conscious experience' in *Experimental and Theoretical Studies of Consciousness.* Ciba Foundation Symposia series, no. 174. Chichester: Wiley, 247–62.

Gilbert, P., Broomhead, C., Irons, C., McEwan, K., Bellew, R., Mills, A., Gale, C. & Knibb, R. (2007). Striving to avoid inferiority: Scale development and its relationship to depression, anxiety and stress. *British Journal of Social Psychology.* **46**, 633–48.

Gilbert, P. & Choden, P. (2014). *Mindful Compassion.* Oakland, California: New Harbinger Publications Ltd.

Goetz, J.L., Keltner, D. & Simon-Thomas, E. (2010). Compassion: An evolutionary analysis and empirical review. *Psychological Bulletin.* **136**, 351–74.

Haith-Cooper, M. (2000). Problem-based learning within health professional education. What is the role of the lecturer? *Nurse Education Today.* **20**, 267–72.

Hallowell, E. (January 2005). Overloaded circuits: Why smart people underperform. *Harvard Business Review.* 55–62.

Hammond, S. & Royal, C. (1998). *Lessons from the Field: Applying Appreciative Inquiry.* Bend, Oregon: Thin Book Publishing Co.

Hart, C. (2000). *Doing a Literature Review. Releasing Social Science Research Imagination.* London: Sage Publications Ltd.

Hasson, G. (2013). *Mindfulness – Be Mindful. Live in the Moment.* Chichester, Sussex: Capstone Publishing Ltd.

Hawkins, D.R. (2006). *Power vs Force – the hidden determinants of human behaviour.* Hay House UK Ltd, London: Her Majesty's Stationery Office.

Hayes, S.C., Strosahl, K., Wilson, K.G., Bissett, R.T., Pistorello, J., Toarmino, D., *et al.* (2004). Measuring experiential avoidance: A preliminary test of a working model. *The Psychological Record*, **54**, 553–78.

HCPC (2014). *Professionalism in healthcare professionals.* HCPC. Pub code MORROW1. London. http://www.hpc-uk.org/assets/documents/10003771Professionalisminhealthcareprofessionals.pdf (accessed 9th November 2014).

Healthcare Commission (2007). *Healthcare Commission Annual Report.* London: The Stationery Office.

Heppner, P., Rogers, M. & Lee, L. (1984). Carl Rogers. Reflections on his life. *Journal of Counselling and Development.* **63**, 14–20

Hohman, M. & Rollnick, S. (2011). *Motivational Interviewing in Social Work Practice.* New York: Guilford Press.

Hornett, M. (2012). Compassionate leadership. *British Journal of Nursing.* **21** (13), 831.

Human Rights Act (1998). http://www.legislation.gov.uk/ukpga/1998/42/contents (Accessed 28 May 2015).

Jackson, S.E. & Dutton, J.E. (1998). Discerning threats and opportunities. *Administrative Science Quarterly.* **33**, 370–87.

Joint Health Select Committee on the Human Rights of Older People in Healthcare (2007). HC Paper 156-1. HC378-1. London: The Stationery Office.

Jung, C.G. (1967). 'Commentary on "The Secret Golden Flower"' in *Collected Works. Vol 13. Alchemical Studies.* London: Routledge and Kegan Paul.

Kabat-Zinn, J. (1994). *Wherever You Go, There You Are: Mindfulness Meditation in Everyday Life.* New York: Hyperion.

Kadushin, A. & Harkness, D. (2002). *Supervision in Social Work* (4th edn). New York: Columbia University Press.

Kanov, J., Maitlis, S., Worline, M.C., Dutton, J.E., Frost, P.J. & Lilius, J. (2004). Compassion in organizational life. *American Behavioural Sciences.* **47**, 808–27

Kennedy Report (2001). The Report of the Public Inquiry into children's heart surgery at the Bristol Royal Infirmary 1984–1995. Public Inquiry. London: The Stationery Office. http://www.wales.nhs.uk/sites3/documents/441/The%20Kennedy%20Report.pdf (Accessed 18 September 2014).

References

Keogh, B. (2013). Review into the quality of care and treatment provided by 14 hospital trusts in England: overview report. London: NHS.

Kirwan, M., Matthews, A. & Scott, P.A. (2013). The impact of the work environment of nurses on patient safety outcomes: A multi-level modelling approach. *International Journal of Nursing Studies*. **50**, 253–63.

Kolb, D. (1984). *Experiential Learning Experience as the Source of Learning and Development*. New Jersey: Prentice Hall.

Kotter, J. (1998). Why transformation efforts fail. *Harvard Business Review of Change*. 1–20.

Lambros, A. (2004). *Problem-based Learning in Middle and High School Classrooms: A teacher's guide to implementation*. Thousand Oaks. California: Corwin Press.

Langer, E. (1989). *Mindfulness*. New York: Perseus Books.

Langer, E. (1997). *The Power of Mindful Learning*. New York: Perseus Books.

Langer, E. (2000). Mindful learning. *Current Directions in Psychological Science*. **9** (6), 220–23.

Langer, E. (2005a). *On Becoming an Artist: Reinventing yourself through mindful creativity*. New York: Ballantine Books.

Langer, E. (2005b). 'Mindfulness versus positive evaluation' in C.R. Snyder & S.J. Lopez (eds). *Handbook of Positive Psychology*. Oxford: Oxford University Press, 214–30.

LeDoux, J.E. (2002). Emotion, memory, and the brain. *Scientific American*. **12**, 62–71.

Lewis, S., Passmore, J. & Cantore, S. (2008). Appreciative enquiry for change management: Using AI to facilitate organisational development. *Industrial and Commercial Training*. **40** (6).

Ludema, J.D., Cooperrider, J.L. & Barrett, F.J. (2006). 'Appreciative Inquiry: the Power of the Unconditional Positive Question' in P. Reason & H. Bradbury (eds). *The Handbook of Action Research*. London: Sage.

Lundahl, B. & Burke, B.L. (2009). The effectiveness and applicability of motivational interviewing: a practice-friendly review of four meta-analyses. *Journal of Clinical Psychology*. **65** (11), 1232–45.

Machon, A. (2005). *Just beyond the Visible – The art of being and becoming*. Croydon, Surrey: Arem Publishing.

Machon, A. (2008). *A Difference of One*. England, UK: Oliver's Books.

Machon, A. (2010). *The Coaching Secret – how to be an exceptional coach*. Harlow, Essex: Pearson Education Ltd.

Machon, A. & Roberts, G.W. (2010). 'An evolving vision of learning in health-care education' in T. Clouston, *et al.* (eds). *Problem based learning in health and social care*. Oxford: Wiley Blackwell, 147–58.

Mayeroff, M. (1971). *On Caring*. New York: HarperCollins.

McKenna, J. & Supyk, J.A. (2006). Using Problem Based Methodology to Develop Reflection as a Core Skill for Undergraduate Students. Conference paper. Problem Based Learning 2004: A Quality Experience Across Boundaries, Across Disciplines and Across the Globe. http://usir.salford.ac.uk (Accessed 22 April 2013).

Mental Health Foundation (2010). Mindfulness Report. p 6. London. Cited by Chaskalson, M. (2011). *The Mindful Workplace – Developing Resilient Individuals and Resonant Organizations with MBSR*. Chichester, Sussex: John Wiley and Sons, Ltd, 3.

Muraven, M., Tice, D. & Baumeister, R.F. (1998). Self-control as a limited resource: Regulatory depletion patterns. *Journal of Personality and Social Psychology*. **74** (3), 774–89.

Murray, E. & Simpson, J. (2000). *Professional Development and Management for Therapists*. Oxford: Blackwell Science.

Najjar, S., Hamdan, M., Euwema, M.C., Vleugels, A., Sermeus, W., Massoud, R. & Vanhaecht, K. (2013). The Global Trigger Tool shows that one out of seven patients suffer harm in Palestinian hospitals: challenges for launching a strategic safety plan. *International Journal for Quality in Healthcare.* **25**, 640–47.

NHS (2013). The NHS Constitution for England, 2013. pp. 3-4. https://www.gov.uk/government/publications/the-nhs-constitution-for-england (Accessed 11 May 2015).

NHS Executive (2013). The 6Cs in Action. http://www.nationalhealthexecutive.com/Featured-Articles/the-6-cs-in-action (Accessed 27 December 2014).

Nordenfelt, L. (2012). *Dignity. Encyclopaedia of Applied Ethics*. Oxford, Elsevier. 800–806.

Nursing and Midwifery Council (2010). *Standards for Pre-registration Nursing Education*. London: NMC.

Nursing and Midwifery Council (2013). NMC response to the Francis Report. The response of the Mid Staffordshire NHS Foundation Trust Public Inquiry report, 18 July 2013. http://www.nmc.org.uk/globalassets/siteDocuments/Francis-report/NMC-response-to-the-Francis-report-18-July.pdf (Accessed 11 May 2015).

Nursing Times (2013). Professionalism is the best regulator of nursing care. http://www.nursingtimes.net/home/specialisms/infection-control/professionalism-is-the-best-regulator-of-nursing-care/5055309.article (Accessed 11 May 2015).

Orem, S.L., Binkert, J. & Clancy, A.L. (2007). *Appreciative Coaching: A Positive Process for Change*. New Jersey: Jossey-Bass.

Ovretveit, J., Mathias, P. & Thompson, T. (1997). *Interprofessional Working for Health and Social Care*. Basingstoke: Macmillan.

Pani, L. (2000). Is there an evolutional mismatch between the normal physiology of the human dopaminergic system and current environmental conditions in industrialised countries? *Molecular Psychiatry.* **5**, 467–75.

Peltier, B. (2010). *The Psychology of Executive Coaching – Theory and Application*. New York: Routledge.

Peterson, C. & Seligman, M.E. (2004). *Character Strengths and Virtues*. New York: Oxford University Press.

Pinder, R.J., Greaves, F.E., Aylin, P.P., Jarman, B. & Bottle, A. (2013). Staff perceptions of quality of care: an observational study of the NHS Staff Survey in hospitals in England. *British Medical Journal of Quality & Safety.* **22**, 563–70.

Polglase, T. & Tresender, R. (2012). *The Occupational Therapy Handbook: Practice Education*. Keswick: M&K Publishing.

Pritchard, J. (2009). *Good Practice in the Law and Safeguarding Adults: Criminal Justice and Adult Protection*. London: Jessica Kingsley Publishers.

Quality Assurance Agency for Higher Education (2007). Code of best practice. http://www.qaa.ac.uk/Pages/default.aspx (Accessed 18 June 2014).

Quinn, F.M. & Hughes, S., (2007). *Quinn's Principles and Practice Nurse Education*. Cheltenham: Nelson Thomas.

Riley, J. & Matheson, R. (2010). 'Promoting creative thinking andinnovative practice through the use of problem based learning' in T. Clouston *et al.* (eds). *Problem Based Learning in Health and Social Care*. Oxford: Wiley Blackwell, 125–38.

References

Roberts, G.W. (2005). 'Aspects of professionalism-factors influencing allied health practice' in T.J. Clouston & L.P. Westcott (eds). *Working in Health and Social Care: An introduction for Allied Health Professionals.* Edinburgh: Elsevier/Churchill Livingstone.

Roberts, G.W. (2010). Advancing new approaches to learning and teaching – introducing appreciative inquiry to a problem-based learning curriculum. *Journal of Applied Research in Higher Education.* **2** (1), 16–24.

Roberts, G.W. (2013). Appreciative inquiry – a new dimension in problem-based learning. *The International HETL Review 2013.* 71–81.

Rollnick W.R. & Miller, S. (2002). *Motivational Interviewing: Preparing people for change.* (2nd edn). New York: Guilford Press.

Rogers, C. (1961). *On Becoming a Person.* Boston: Houghton Mifflin.

Rogers, C. (1983). *Freedom to Learn in the 80's.* Ohio: Charles Merrill Publishing Co.

Roseneder, S., Lancee, J. & Crowder, R. (2004). PBL Stories and Signposts. ENOTHE – World Federation of Occupational Therapists. Hogeschool Amsterdam.one. 103–13.

Ross, J. (2011). Patient safety outcomes: The importance of understanding the organizational culture and safety climate. *Journal of PeriAnesthesia Nursing.* **26**, 347–48.

Ross, L. & McSherry, W. (2010). 'Considerations for the future of spiritual assessment' in W. McSherry & L. Ross (eds). *Spiritual Assessment in Healthcare Practice.* Keswick: M&K Publishing, 162.

Royal College of Nursing (2008). *Defending Dignity – Challenges and Opportunities for Nursing.* London: RCN. http://www.rcn.org.uk/publications. (Accessed 19 April 2014).

Rubin, R., Kerrell, R. & Roberts, G.W. (2011). Appreciative inquiry in occupational therapy education. *British Journal of Occupational Therapy.* **74** (5), 233–40.

Sachs, J. (2011). *The Price of Civilisation: Economics and Ethics After the Fall.* London: Bodley.

Sadlo, G. (2004). 'Creativity and Occupation' in M. Molineux (ed). *Occupation for Occupational Therapists.* Oxford: Blackwell Publishers.

Savin-Baden, M. & Major, C.H. (2004). *Foundations of Problem-based Learning.* Buckingham: SRHE. Open University Press.

Seligman, M.E.P. (2002). *Authentic Happiness.* New York: Free Press.

Seligman, M.E.P. & Maier, S.F. (1967). Failure to escape traumatic shock. *Journal of Experimental Psychology.* **74**, 1–9.

Seligman, M.E.P. & Csikszentmihalyi, M. (2000). Positive psychology: An introduction. *American Psychologist.* **55** (1), 5–14.

Siegel, D.J. (2007). *The Mindful Brain.* New York: Norton.

Social Care Institute for Excellence (2010). http://www.scie.org.uk/publications/guides/guide15/index.asp (Accessed 31 June 2012).

Standal, W.S. (1954). *The Need for Positive Regard: A Contribution to Client-centred Therapy.* Chicago: University of Chicago, Department of Psychology Publications.

Stantham, D. (2000). Guest editorial: Partnership between health and social care. *Health and Social Care in the Community.* **8**, 87–89.

Starfield, B. (2011). Is patient-centered care the same as person-focused care? *The Permanente Journal.* **15** (2), 63–69.

Synder, C.R. & Ingram, R.E. (2006). Special issue on positive psychology. *Journal of Cognitive Psychotherapy: An International Quarterly.* **20**, 115–240.

Tadd, W. & Bayer, A. (2006). Dignity in health and social care for older Europeans: Implications of a European project. *Aging Health.* **2** (5), 771–79.

Tadd, W. & Calnan, M. (2009). 'Caring for Older People: Why Dignity Matters - The European Experience' in I. Nordenfelt (ed). *Dignity in Care for Older People.* Oxford: Wiley-Blackwell, 119–42.

Taylor, M.B. (1997). Compassion: Its neglect and importance. *British Journal of General Practice.* **47**, 521–23.

Worth, P. (2000). *Localised Creativity. A Lifespan Perspective.* Milton Keynes: Open University.

Upton, D., Stephens, D., Williams, B. & Scurlock-Evans, L. (2014). Occupational therapists' attitudes, knowledge and implementation of evidence-based practice: a systematic review of published research. *British Journal of Occupational Therapy.* **77** (1), 24–38.

You, L.M., Aiken, L.H., Sloane, D.M., Liu, K., He, G.-P., Hu,Y., Jiang, X.-L., LI, X.-H., LI,X.-M., Liu, H.-P., Shang, S.-M., Kutney-Lee, A. & Sermeus, W. (2013). Hospital nursing, care quality, and patient satisfaction: Cross-sectional surveys of nurses and patients in hospitals in China and Europe. *International Journal of Nursing Studies.* **50**, 154–61.

Weick. K.E. & Putnam, T. (2006). Organizing for mindfulness: Eastern Wisdom and Western Knowledge. *Journal of Management Inquiry.* **15** (3), 275–87.

Weiner, S.J. & Auster, S. (2007). From empathy to caring: defining the ideal approach to a healing relationship. *Yale Journal of Biology and Medicine.* **80** (3) 123–27.

Whiteford, G. & Wilcock, A. (2002). Cultural relativism: occupation and culture reconsidered. Canadian *Journal of Occupational Therapy.* 67 (5), 324–36.

Whitmore, J. (2004). *Coaching for Performance – Growing People, Performance and Purpose.* London: Nicholas Brealey Publishing.

Williams, M., Teasdale, J., Segal, S. & Kabat-Zinn, J. (2007). *The Mindful Way Through Depression: Freeing Yourself from Chronic Unhappiness.* London: Guilford Press.

Bibliography

Addicott, R. & Ashton, R. eds. (2010). *Delivering Better Care at End of Life: The next steps.* London: The King's Fund.

Agich, G.J. (2007). Reflections on the function of dignity in the context of caring for old people. *Journal of Medicine and Philosophy.* **32** (5), 483–94.

Alzheimer's Society (2009). *Counting the Cost: Caring for people with dementia on hospital wards.* London: Alzheimer's Society.

Anderberg, P., Lepp, M., Berglund, A.L. & Segesten, K. (2007). Preserving dignity in caring for older adults: a concept analysis. *Journal of Advanced Nursing.* **59** (6), 635–43.

Andersson, M., Hallberg, I.R. & Edberg, A.K. (2008). Old people receiving municipal care, their experiences of what constitutes a good life in the last phase of life: a qualitative study. *International Journal of Nursing Studies.* **45** (6), 818–28.

Arino-Blasco, S., Tadd, W. & Boix-Ferrer, J.A. (2005). Dignity and older people. *Quality in Ageing: Policy Practice and Research.* **6**, 30–36.

Audit Commission (2004). *Older people – independence and well-being: the challenge for public services.* London: Audit Commission.

Baillie, L. (2008). Mixed-sex wards and patient dignity: nurses' and patients' perspectives. *British Journal of Nursing.* **17** (19), 1220–225.

Baillie, L. (2009). Patient dignity in an acute hospital setting: a case study. *International Journal of Nursing Studies.* **46** (1), 23–36.

Barnes, M., Blom, A., Cox, K., Lessof, C. & Walker, A. (2006). *New horizons: The social exclusion of older people: secondary analysis of the English longitudinal study of ageing.* National Centre for Social Research and University of Sheffield.

Bayer, T., Tadd, W. & Krajcik, S. (2005). Dignity: the voice of older people. *Quality in Ageing: Policy Practice and Research.* **6**, 22–29.

Bowles, M.L. (1991). The organization shadow. *Organization Studies.* **12** (3), 387.

Bushe, G.R. (2007a). Generativity and the transformational potential of appreciative inquiry. *Organizational Generativity: Advances in Appreciative Inquiry.* 3.

Bushe, G.R. (2007b). Appreciative inquiry is not (just) about the positive. *OD Practitioner.* **39** (4), 30–35.

Chochinov, H. M., Hack, T., Hassard, T., Kristjanson, L.J., Mcclement, S. & Harlos, M. (2002a). Dignity in the terminally ill: a cross-sectional, cohort study. *The Lancet.* **360**, 2026–2030.

Chochinov, H. M., Hack, T., Mcclement, S., Kristjanson, L.J. & Harlos, M. (2002b). Dignity in the terminally ill: a developing empirical model. *Social Science and Medicine.* **54**, 433–43.

Chochinov, H. (2007). Dignity and the essence of medicine – the A, B, C, and D of dignity conserving care. *British Medical Journal.* **335** (7612), 184–87.

Chochinov, H.M. (2006). Dying, dignity, and new horizons in palliative end-of-life care. CA: a Cancer *Journal for Clinicians.* **56** (2), 84–103.

Chochinov, H.M. *et al.* (2006). Dignity in the terminally ill: revisited. *Journal of Palliative Medicine.* **9** (3), 666–72.

Chochinov, H.M., Hassard, T., McClement, S. (2008). The patient dignity inventory: a novel way of measuring dignity-related distress in palliative care. *Journal of Pain and Symptom Management.* **36** (6), 559–71.

Cooperrider, D. L. & S. Srivastva (1987). Appreciative inquiry in organizational life, in R. Woodman and W. Pasmore (eds). *Research in Organizational Change and Development.* **1**, 129–69. Greenwich, CT: JAI Press Inc.

Cooperrider, D.L. & Barrett, F.J. (2002). An Exploration of the Spiritual Heart of Human Science Inquiry. *Reflections.* **3** (3), 56–62.

Donovan, L.L., Meyer, S.R. & Fitzgerald, S.P. (2007a). Transformative Learning and Appreciative Inquiry: A More Perfect Union for Deep Organizational Change. Academy of Management Proceedings, Columbia University Teachers College.

Donovan, L.L., Meyer, S.R. & Fitzgerald, S.P. (2007b). Transformative Learning and Appreciative Inquiry: A More Perfect Union for Deep Organizational Change. Academy of Management Proceedings, Columbia University Teachers College, 4.

Grant, S. & Humphries, M. (2006). Critical evaluation of appreciative inquiry: Bridging an apparent paradox. *Action Research.* **4** (4).

Jessop, T. (2009). Dangerous dreams: the change potential of appreciative inquiry. HEIR Network Conference Proceedings, University of Worcester.

Kelm, J.B. (2005). Appreciative Living: The Principles of Appreciative Inquiry in Personal Life. http://www.AppreciativeLiving.com (Accessed 12 May 2015).

Landsberg, M. (2003). *The Tao of Coaching: Boost your effectiveness at work by inspiring and developing those around you.* London: Profile Books.

Lewin, K. (1951). *Field Theory in Social Science.* New York: Harper and Row.

Lovallo, D. & D. Kahneman (2003). Delusions of success: How optimism undermines executives' decisions. *Harvard Business Review.* **81** (7), 56–63.

Liebling, A., Price, D. & Elliott, C. (1999). Appreciative inquiry and relationships in prison. *Punishment and Society.* **1** (1).

Ludema, J.D., Cooperrider, D.L. & Barrett, F.J. (2006). 'Appreciative Inquiry: the Power of the Unconditional Positive Question' in P. Reason & H. Bradbury (eds). *The Handbook of Action Research.* New York: Sage.

Peters, S. (2012). *The Chimp Paradox – The Mind Management Programme for Confidence, Success and Happiness.* London: Vermilion, Random House.

Rogers, P.J. & Fraser, D. (Winter 2003). Appreciating Appreciative Inquiry. *New Directions for Evaluation.* (100), 75–83.

Sadlo, G. (2004). 'Creativity and Occupation' in M. Molineux (ed). *Occupation for Occupational Therapists.* Oxford: Blackwell.

Salopek, J.J. (August 2006). Appreciative Inquiry at 20: Questioning David Cooperrider. *Trends.* **60** (8), 21

Savin-Baden, M. & Major, C.H (2004). *Foundations of problem based learning.* Buckingham: SRHE. Open University Press.

Social Exclusion Unit and Office of the Deputy Prime Minister (2006). A sure start to later life: ending inequalities for older people: final report. London: Social Exclusion Unit.

References

Springfield, F. (2002). Lesbians, gays and transsexuals in care homes. *Nursing and Residential Care.* **4**, 586–88.

Stratton, D. & Tadd, W. (2005). Dignity and older people: the voice of society. *Quality in Ageing: Policy Practice and Research.* **6**, 37–45.

Street, A. F. & Love, A. (2005). Dimensions of privacy in palliative care: views of health professionals. *Social Science and Medicine.* **60**, 1795–1804.

Van der Haar, D. & Hosking, D.M. (2004). Evaluating appreciativeinquiry: A relational constructionist perspective. *Human Relations.* **57** (8).

Wineburg, S.S. (1987). The self-fulfillment of the self-fulfilling prophesy. *Educational Researcher.* **16** (9).

Wright, M. & Baker, A. (2005). The effects of appreciative inquiry interviews on staff in the UK National Health Service. *International Journal of Healthcare Quality Assurance.* **18** (1), 41–45.